Anaesthesia
on the move

Anaesthesia
on the move

Authors: **Sally Keat, Simon Townend Bate, Alexander Bown and Sarah Lanham**
Editorial Advisor: **Peter Matthews**
Series Editors: **Rory Mackinnon, Sally Keat, Thomas Locke and Andrew Walker**

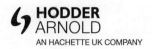
HODDER
ARNOLD
AN HACHETTE UK COMPANY

First published in Great Britain in 2012 by
Hodder Arnold, an imprint of Hodder Education, a division of Hachette UK
338 Euston Road, London NW1 3BH

http://www.hodderarnold.com

Whilst the advice and information in this book are believed to be true and accurate at the date of going to press, neither the author[s] nor the publisher can accept any legal responsibility or liability for any errors or omissions that may be made. In particular, (but without limiting the generality of the preceding disclaimer) every effort has been made to check drug dosages; however, it is still possible that errors have been missed. Furthermore, dosage schedules are constantly being revised and new side-effects recognized. For these reasons the reader is strongly urged to consult the drug companies' printed instructions, and their websites, before administering any of the drugs recommended in this book.

British Library Cataloguing in Publication Data
A catalogue record for this book is available from the British Library

Library of Congress Cataloging-in-Publication Data
A catalog record for this book is available from the Library of Congress

ISBN-13   978-1-444-12153-7

1 2 3 4 5 6 7 8 9 10
Commissioning Editor: Joanna Koster
Project Editor: Stephen Clausard
Production Controller: Francesca Wardell
Cover Design: Amina Dudhia
Indexer: Laurence Errington

Cover image © LTH NHS Trust/Science Photo Library
Typeset in 10/12 pt Adobe Garamond Pro Regular by Datapage
Printed and bound in India by Replika Press

What do you think about this book? Or any other Hodder Arnold title?
Please visit our website: www.hodderarnold.com

Contents

Preface

Anaesthesia is an exciting, rapidly changing specialty. It is loved by students for its practical nature and reputation as being at the sharp end of patient care. Anaesthetics is also inextricably linked with physiology and pharmacology. This makes it an ideal topic to help bridge the gap between basic sciences and clinical medicine. Written by students for students, this short guide to anaesthetics also gives a whirlwind tour of human physiology. We aimed to give information in as many different styles as possible, keeping the text engaging. We hope this brief guide will give you: the tools to handle an emergency situation, the ablity to optimise a patient both peri-operatively and on the ward and, most importantly (!), withstand a grilling on your anaesthetics placement.

AUTHORS:

Sally Keat BMedSci MBChB – Foundation Year 1 doctor, Northern General Hospital, Sheffield, UK

Simon Townend Bate BMedSci MBChB – Foundation Year 1 doctor, Barnsley Hospital, UK

Alexander Bown MBChB – Foundation Year 2 doctor, Sheffield Teaching Hospitals, UK

Sarah Lanham MBChB – Foundation Year 2 doctor, Sheffield Teaching Hospitals, UK

EDITORIAL ADVISOR:

Peter Matthews – Consultant Anaesthetist, Rotherham NHS Foundation Trust, Rotherham, UK

EDITOR-IN-CHIEF

Rory Mackinnon BSc MBChB – Foundation Year 2 doctor, Northern General Hospital, Sheffield, UK

SERIES EDITORS:

Sally Keat BMedSci MBChB – Foundation Year 1 doctor, Northern General Hospital, Sheffield, UK

Thomas Locke BSc MBChB – Foundation Year 1 doctor, Northern General Hospital, Sheffield, UK

Andrew Walker BMedSci MBChB – Specialist Trainee Year 1 doctor in Medicine, Chesterfield Royal Hospital, Chesterfield, Derbyshire, UK

Acknowledgements

The authors would like to thank Pete Matthews for being hugely helpful during the writing of this book and for supplying the photographs.

We would also like to thank Chesterfield Royal Hospital for kindly allowing us to use their anaesthetic charts and questionnaires as example material.

List of abbreviations

- ABG: arterial blood gas
- ACE: angiotensin-converting enzyme
- ACh: acetylcholine
- ADH: anti-diuretic hormone
- AKI: acute kidney injury
- ASA: American Society of Anaesthesiologists
- ASV: assisted spontaneous ventilation
- ATP: adenosine triphosphate
- AV: atrioventricular
- BD: two times daily
- BiPAP: bilevel positive airways pressure
- BMI: body mass index
- BP: blood pressure
- CN: cranial nerve
- CNS: central nervous system
- COPD: chronic obstructive pulmonary disease
- COX: cyclo-oxygenase
- CPAP: continuous positive airway pressure
- CPP: cerebral perfusion pressure
- CSF: cerebrospinal fluid
- CTZ: chemoreceptor trigger zone
- CVA: cerebrovascular accident
- CVP: central venous pressure
- CVVH: continuous venovenous haemofiltration
- D_2: dopamine
- DBP: diastolic blood pressure
- DKA: diabetic ketoacidosis
- DM: diabetes mellitus
- DVT: deep vein thrombosis
- ECF: extra-cellular fluid
- ECG: echocardiogram
- EDV: end-diastolic volume
- ERV: expiratory reserve volume
- ESV: end-systolic volume
- ET: endotracheal
- EWS: early warning scoring
- FBC: full blood count
- FiO_2: fraction of inspired O_2
- FRC: functional residual capacity

- GA: general anaesthetic
- GCS: Glasgow Coma Scale
- GI: gastrointestinal
- GIK: glucose–insulin–potassium
- Hb: haemoglobin
- HDU: high dependency unit
- HR: heart rate
- HRS: hepatorenal syndrome
- IHD: ischaemic heart disease
- IL: interleukin
- IM: intramuscular
- INR: international normalized ratio
- IPPV: intermittent positive pressure ventilation
- IRV: inspiratory reserve volume
- ITU: intensive therapy unit
- IV: intravenous
- JVP: jugular venous pressure
- LAP: left atrial pressure
- LMA: laryngeal mask airway
- LMWH: low molecular weight heparin
- LV: left ventricle
- LVEDU: left ventricle end-diastolic volume
- LVF: left ventricular function
- MAC: mean alveolar concentration
- MAP: mean arterial pressure
- MI: myocardial infarction
- MMT: modified Mallampatti technique
- N_2O: nitrous oxide
- nAChR: nicotinic acetylcholine receptor
- NE: noradrenaline
- NIPPV: non-invasive positive pressure ventilation
- NIV: non-invasive ventilation
- NMB: neuromuscular blocker
- NRB: non-rebreathe
- NSAIDs: non-steroidal anti-inflammatory drugs
- NT: nasotracheal
- *P*: (partial) pressure
- PCA: patient controlled analgesia
- PE: pulmonary embolism
- PEEP: positive end-expiratory pressure
- PEFR: peak expiratory flow rate
- PONV: post-operative nausea and vomiting
- PP: pulse pressure

- PTH: parathyroid hormone
- PVR: peripheral vascular resistance
- *Q*: perfusion
- QDS: four times daily
- RA: rheumatoid arthritis
- RBC: red blood cell
- RR: respiratory rate
- RSI: rapid sequence induction
- RTI: respiratory tract infection
- RV: right ventricle/residual volume
- *S*: saturation
- SA: sinoatrial
- SBP: systolic blood pressure
- SIADH: syndrome of inappropriate anti-diuretic hormone secretion
- SIMV: synchronized intermittent mandatory ventilation
- SIRS: systemic inflammatory response syndrome
- SV: stroke volume
- TDS: three times daily
- TENS: transcutaneous electrical nerve stimulation
- TLC: total lung capacity
- TV: tidal volume
- U&Es: urea and electrolytes
- URTI: upper respiratory tract infection
- *V*: ventilation
- VC: vital capacity
- WPW: Wolff–Parkinson–White syndrome

An explanation of the text

The book is divided into five parts, which aim to divide anaesthesia into sections loosely following a journey from pre-assessment to surgery and back to the wards. We have used bullet points to keep the text concise, supplementing this with diagrams, flowcharts and photographs. MICRO-boxes are dotted throughout (explained below).

We have included a brief formulary of common anaesthetic drugs. This is in no way exhaustive, but can be used to gain an understanding of the classes of drugs used in anaesthesia. Doses are not given, as these vary widely according to local protocols. The most up-to-date practices and therapies have been included, but always check local guidelines for current practice.

> ## MICRO-facts
> These boxes expand on the text and contain clinically relevant facts and memorable summaries of the essential information.

> ## MICRO-print
> These boxes contain additional information to the text that may interest certain readers but is not essential for everybody to learn.

> ## MICRO-case
> These boxes contain clinical cases relevant to the text and include a number of summary bullet points to highlight the key learning objectives.

> ## MICRO-techniques
> These boxes contain step-by-step guides to useful procedures, most of which are essential skills for junior doctors.

> ## MICRO-reference
> These boxes contain references to important clinical research and national guidance.

Part Ⅰ

Pre-operative

1 Physiology

Anaesthetists modulate human physiology. This means that:

- to have a broad understanding of the principles of anaesthetics, you must first have an overview of relevant physiology;
- during anaesthesia you are able to observe an immediate and measurable effect on physiology after administering drugs;
- pharmacology is also hugely important to the practice of anaesthesia and is better understood when thought of in terms of action on human physiology.

1.1 HOMEOSTASIS

Anaesthetists aim to maintain homeostasis. The following section will cover important aspects of homeostasis, in relation to anaesthesia.

Homeostasis is the ability of an organic system to maintain internal equilibrium by adjusting physiological processes. These processes are reversible changes which maintain a stable internal environment.

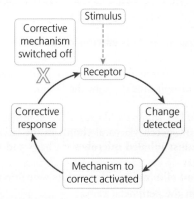

Fig. 1.1 Homeostatic mechanism.

CONTROL OF HOMEOSTASIS

- Homeostasis is largely controlled by **negative feedback loops**. These involve:
    - an increase or decrease of a particular variable;
    - activation of a chain of events that opposes the change in the variable;
    - a return of the variable to normal levels.
- Attributes of negative feedback mechanisms are:
    - prevention of large deviations from the normal range;
    - relatively small deviations trigger a feedback mechanism.
- Negative feedback can originate at a molecular, cellular or organ level.
- The product formed often inhibits the initial enzyme in the homeostatic mechanism.
- Examples of negative feedback loops include the control of blood sugar, temperature and blood pressure (BP).

MICRO-print
- **Positive feedback** occurs only in certain situations.
- Positive feedback is designed to enhance a process which has already been stimulated and to drive the variable to go out of the normal range.
- An example is the posterior pituitary hormone oxytocin, produced in response to uterine stretching at the start of labour. Production of oxytocin induces further contractions, which further stretches the uterus, promoting the production of oxytocin. This causes a rapid escalation of hormone-controlled contractions leading to the birth of the baby.

1.2 RESPIRATORY PHYSIOLOGY

ROLE OF THE RESPIRATORY SYSTEM

- The respiratory system controls **gaseous exchange**.
- This involves:
    - oxygenating the blood and therefore supplying tissues within the body;
    - removal of carbon dioxide from the blood.
- It is also involved in:
    - **regulation of H^+** within the blood and therefore maintenance of blood pH;
    - **formation of speech** via vocal chords in the larynx;
    - **defence against inhaled microbes** via hairs and mucous in the nasopharynx;
    - **trapping and eliminating blood clots** sent into circulation after formation in the peripheral veins;
    - **production of angiotensin-converting enzyme**, which cleaves angiotensin I to form angiotensin II.

MECHANISM OF BREATHING

Respiratory organization

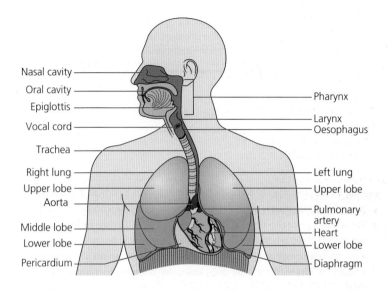

Nasal cavity

Oral cavity

Epiglottis

Vocal cord

Trachea

Right lung

Upper lobe

Aorta

Middle lobe

Lower lobe

Pericardium

Pharynx

Larynx

Oesophagus

Left lung

Upper lobe

Pulmonary artery

Heart

Lower lobe

Diaphragm

Fig. 1.2 **Anatomy of the respiratory system.**

- Gas exchange occurs in the alveoli:
  - Alveoli contain **type I** and **type II** pneumocytes. These cells are roughly the same in number but type I make up over 95% of the surface area:
    - Type I: flat epithelial cells which make up the thin (0.2 μm) wall of the alveolus. The thin wall minimizes the distance for gas to diffuse across, maximizing gas exchange to the capillaries surrounding the alveolus.
    - Type II: produce surfactant, which lowers surface tension. These cells are dotted in between type I cells.
- Ventilation is achieved by the relationship between the lungs and the thoracic wall:
  - The intercostal muscles, ribs, sternum and spinal column make up the walls of the thorax, with the diaphragm separating the thorax from the abdomen below.
  - The lungs are attached to the thoracic wall via the pleurae. The pleurae are two parts of a folded membrane; the visceral pleura overlies the lungs and the parietal pleura overlies the thoracic wall and diaphragm.
  - Pressure gradients needed to force air into and out of the lungs are created by these relationships.

> **MICRO-print**
> **Boyle's law** explains why the change in lung dimensions (inspiration = chest wall moving out and the diaphragm moving down, which are reversed on expiration) affects the flow of gas: $P_1V_1 = P_2V_2$.
>   This equation represents that the pressure (P) exerted by a gas is inversely proportional to the volume (V) of the container.

Lung mechanics

- **Ventilation** is the exchange of air between the atmosphere and lungs.
- Air flows from areas of high pressure to areas of low pressure.
- Air flow can be calculated by:

$$F = (P_{alv} - P_{atm})/R$$

  where F is flow, P_{alv} is alveolar pressure (always given as relative to atmospheric pressure), P_{atm} is atmospheric pressure (pressure outside the body and within the mouth and nose) and R is airway resistance.
- This means that, when air flows into the lungs, it is because alveolar pressure is less than atmospheric pressure. The reverse is true on expiration.
- Changes in alveolar pressure are caused by changes in transpulmonary pressure and stretching of the lungs:
  - Transpulmonary pressure depends upon:
    - the pressure inside the lungs (alveolar pressure) and the pressure outside the lungs (intra-pleural fluid pressure);
    - it can be represented as:

$$P_{tp} = P_{alv} - P_{ip}$$

    where P_{tp} is the transpulmonary pressure and P_{ip} is the intra-pleural fluid pressure.

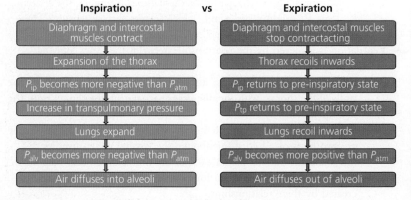

Fig. 1.3 Processes occuring during inspiration and expiration.

Lung compliance and resistance

Compliance

- **Compliance** (stretchability) can be represented as:

$$C_L = \Delta V_L / \Delta(P_{alv} - P_{ip})$$

  where C_L is the compliance of the lungs, ΔV_L is the change in lung volume and $\Delta(P_{alv} - P_{ip})$ is the change in alveolar pressure minus intra-pleural pressure.
- The greater the compliance of the lungs, the more they are able to stretch and therefore more easily move air in and out.
- Compliance is determined by:
  - The **elasticity** of the connective tissue components within the lung, e.g. in **pulmonary fibrosis** the connective tissue is less elastic and stretchable and therefore air flow is reduced.
  - **Surface tension** within the alveoli:
    - As alveoli are lined with water, there is a gas–water interface, the surface of which is maintained by the force of attraction between water molecules or surface tension.
    - Surface tension prevents collapse of the lungs (atelectasis) and subsequent filling with interstitial fluid.
    - **Surfactant** decreases the surface tension making lung expansion easier.
  - **Volume of gas inspired**: at low volumes, compliance is poor owing to the effort required to initiate expansion. With high volumes, poor compliance is observed because of the limits of chest wall movement.

MICRO-facts

Surfactant not only decreases surface tension but also **stabilizes alveoli**. Alveoli differ in size; if all alveoli had the same degree of surface tension, smaller alveoli would have a higher internal pressure and therefore air would preferentially flow into bigger alveoli, causing the small ones to collapse. Surfactant prevents this as its molecules will be more densely packed in small alveoli and therefore the surface tension is decreased. The lower surface tension will increase the internal pressure (according to the **law of Laplace**) and resist collapse.

MICRO-print

Surfactant production by type II alveolar cells is provoked by deep breaths rather than shallow ones. This is why normal breathing at rest mainly consists of shallow breathing, with deep breaths every so often.

continued...

Pre-operative

continued...

This is also one reason post-operative patients who may have reason to use only shallow breathing (such as after abdominal surgery) should be encouraged to take deep breaths when they can. Otherwise, lung compliance will decrease, breathing will be restricted and risk of infection is increased.

Resistance

- Airways resistance:
  - is determined by the **length** of the vessel, vessel **radius** and the **interactions** between the gaseous molecules within the vessel;
  - the most important of these factors is the **vessel radius**.
- Airways resistance to the flow of air is usually very low, which allows small pressure differences to create a large flow of air.
- The vessel radius can be affected by:
  - **transpulmonary pressure**: this is high during inspiration, and opens and distends the non-cartilaginous airways, reducing resistance;
  - **lateral traction**: this is a force created by the connection between the outside edges of the airways and the surrounding alveolar tissue; this reduces resistance by distending the airways during inspiration;
  - **hormones**: these are able to affect airway radii. Activation of the β_2 (and to a lesser extent α_1) adrenergic receptors relaxes smooth muscle of the airways. Leukotrienes increase resistance by causing airway smooth muscle contraction.
- Factors which can affect resistance:
  - **Asthma**:
    - Asthma is characterized by contraction of the smooth muscle of the airways, increasing resistance. The increase in resistance is **reversible**.
    - The contraction is usually triggered by certain substances or conditions, such as smoke, pollen and cold air.
  - **Chronic obstructive pulmonary disease (COPD)**:
    - COPD is characterized by **irreversible** increased resistance. The term collectively describes chronic bronchitis and emphysema:
      - ○ **Chronic bronchitis** is chronic inflammatory change to the mucous membranes of bronchi, causing increased production of mucous.
      - ○ **Emphysema** is the destruction of tissues around the alveoli.
    - These conditions are usually a result of cigarette smoking and result in an increase in airway resistance.

RESPIRATORY VOLUMES

Figure 1.4 shows the lung volumes of a man during breathing at rest, measured by spirometry.

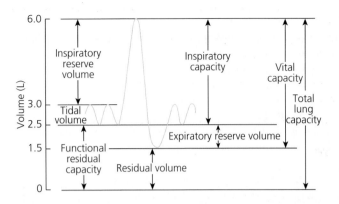

Fig. 1.4 Spirometry graph.

- **Tidal volume** (TV; approximately 0.5 L):
    - the volume of air entering the lungs during a single normal inspiration;
    - the tidal volume multiplied by the respiratory rate gives the **minute volume**.
- **Inspiratory reserve volume** (IRV; up to 3 L):
    - the extra volume of air that can be inspired with maximal effort after reaching the end of a normal, quiet inspiration.
- **Functional residual capacity** (FRC; approximately 2.4 L):
    - the volume of air left in the lungs after normal expiration;
    - this means that the fresh, inspired air is mixing with a reservoir already in the lungs.
- **Expiratory reserve volume** (ERV; 1.2 L):
    - the volume of air which can be expired on maximal expiration when actively using the expiratory muscles.
- **Residual volume** (RV):
    - the volume of air left in the lungs after maximal expiration (FRC–ERV);
    - allows alveoli to stay inflated between breaths.
- **Vital capacity** (VC; 4.7 L):
    - the maximum volume of air which can be expired after maximal inspiration;
    - can be used to assess the strength of the respiratory muscles and lung function.
- **Total lung capacity** (TLC; 6 L):
    - maximum volume the lungs can contain (VC + RV).

Dead space

The concept of dead space within the respiratory system helps to explain the importance of alveolar ventilation as only air which enters the alveoli can take part in gaseous exchange.

- **Anatomical dead space**:
  - 500 mL of air is forced out of the alveoli during each expiration, only 350 mL of this is completely expelled;
  - this leaves 150 mL remaining in the larger airways;
  - during inspiration, a full 500 mL can pass into the alveoli, but 150 mL of this will be the air not previously expired.
- **Alveolar dead space**:
  - not all air that reaches the alveoli takes part in gaseous exchange, owing to perfusion inequalities or pathology;
  - this volume is very small in healthy individuals, but can be significant in those with respiratory diseases affecting the alveoli.
- **Physiological dead space = anatomical dead space + alveolar dead space.**
- **Alveolar ventilation per inspiration = tidal volume − dead space.**

Alveolar ventilation

- Definition:

$$V_A = (V_t - V_D) \times RR$$

where V_A is the alveolar ventilation (mL/min), V_t is the tidal volume (mL/breath), V_D is the dead space (mL/breath) and **RR** is the respiratory rate (breaths/min).

- Alveolar ventilation gives a much better approximation of a person's true ventilation than minute ventilation:
  - smaller, more frequent breaths will produce a minute ventilation similar to that of less regular, deeper breaths. However, a higher proportion of small breaths are taken up by anatomical dead space, reducing the amount of air reaching the alveoli.

Gas exchange

- **Partial pressure**: the pressure a gas would exert if alone in a vessel (which remains the same even if there is a mixture of gases occupying a single vessel):
  - The partial pressure (P) of a gas affects the speed at which it diffuses and dissolves, independent of the concentration.
  - Normal alveolar partial pressures:
    - O_2 − 13.5 kPa;
    - CO_2 − 5 kPa.

MICRO-print
Dalton's law states that the total pressure of a gaseous mixture is equal to the sum of the partial pressures of the individual gases.

- Venous blood circulates around alveoli from pulmonary arteries:
  - This is low in oxyhaemoglobin and high in carboxyhaemoglobin.
  - It creates a concentration gradient, down which O_2 can diffuse into the blood and CO_2 diffuses out. Therefore capillary blood contains similar concentrations of O_2 and CO_2 to alveolar air.
  - Gas exchange is efficient because:
    - Diffusion of gases occurs very quickly (O_2 does not diffuse as well as CO_2, especially at low partial pressures, but this is compensated for by strong binding to haemoglobin (Hb)).
    - Blood in capillaries moves slowly around alveoli.
    - Alveoli have a huge surface area for diffusion.

Ventilation and perfusion

MICRO-facts

West zones divide the lungs up anatomically according to the pressure of the arteries, veins and alveoli. There are **three** zones. The top zone has good ventilation, but poor perfusion. In the middle zone both are good. The lower zone has good perfusion but poor ventilation.

- In healthy individuals ventilation (V) and perfusion (Q) are well matched:
  - When erect, lung bases are better perfused but not as well ventilated as the apices.
  - Because Q falls more than V from base to apex, the apex has a higher V/Q ratio than the base and vice versa. Optimal V/Q is usually in the lower middle zones.
- Ventilation–perfusion mismatch (V/Q mismatch):
  - occurs when the blood flow to the alveoli and rate of gas exchange do not correlate; usually results in a low O_2 concentration in arterial blood;
  - CO_2 can also be raised in severe V/Q mismatch but to a much smaller degree (as CO_2 is 20 times more soluble than O_2).
- V/Q mismatch can be caused by:
  - **Ventilation problems**:
    - Anything that increases resistance, reduces compliance or increases dead space will reduce ventilation capacity. Examples include: interstitial fibrosis, emphysema, COPD and pulmonary oedema.
  - **Perfusion problems**:
    - Limited blood flow will reduce perfusion. Examples include: pulmonary embolus, heart failure.

Pre-operative

MICRO-facts

V/Q mismatching is common in anaesthesia, as the forced vital capacity is greatly reduced in the unconscious patient. Two main types of V/Q mismatch occur.

- **Ventilation of alveolar dead space**
  - This occurs when non-perfused alveoli receive O_2 which cannot be exchanged.
  - Increasing the percentage of O_2 provided will not affect this.
- **Shunt**
  - This occurs when an area of lung which is collapsed or blocked is still perfused, but there is no O_2 to diffuse across.
  - This can be corrected by providing pressure support to re-inflate sections of lung (see Chapter 4, Airways and ventilation).

- Homeostatic mechanisms to prevent severe V/Q mismatch:
  - Alveoli with reduced O_2 prompt the surrounding pulmonary capillaries to vasoconstrict. This diverts blood away from the blocked or diseased alveoli to areas with more O_2 available.
  - Decreased blood flow will cause decreased CO_2 supply, leading to bronchoconstriction and diversion of airflow to better perfused sections of lung.

O_2 and CO_2 transportation in blood

Oxygen

- O_2 is relatively insoluble:
  - Therefore the majority must be bound to another molecule to circulate.
  - This compound is Hb, which consists of:
    - four haem groups, each with an attached polypeptide;
    - haem contains iron, which is able to bind O_2.
  - The amount of O_2-saturated Hb is affected by the PO_2, shown graphically by the oxygen dissociation curve (Fig. 1.5).
  - The affinity of Hb for O_2 increases when the PO_2 is between 20 mmHg and 60 mmHg and then plateaus.
  - The dissociation curve demonstrates how, in areas of high PO_2, Hb will bind O_2, while, in areas of low PO_2, O_2 becomes unbound and diffuses into the tissues.
    - If the affinity of Hb for O_2 is too high, then respiring tissues will not receive O_2, even when saturated Hb circulates through.

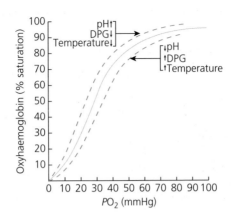

Fig. 1.5 Oxygen dissociation curve. DPG, 2,3-diphosphoglycerate.

- The plateau phase allows for a drop in PO_2 with no effect on Hb saturation. However, several factors can affect the affinity of Hb for O_2:
  - temperature;
  - pH/PCO_2 (Bohr effect);
  - 2,3-diphosphoglycerate produced by red blood cells;
  - carbon monoxide (CO outcompetes O_2 binding because of a higher Hb affinity and also shifts dissociation of O_2 to the left, resulting in O_2 remaining bound rather than being delivered to tissues).

Carbon dioxide
- CO_2 is much more soluble than O_2 and is able to dissolve into blood.
- Around 200 mL CO_2 is produced per minute by metabolism at rest.
- Unlike O_2, CO_2 is carried in the blood in several ways:
  - because of its solubility, a small fraction will dissolve directly into plasma;
  - some will react with Hb to create carboxyhaemoglobin;
  - however, most will react with water in the presence of carbonic anhydrase to create bicarbonate (Fig. 1.6).

Control of ventilation

Ventilation is achieved by a pathway consisting of:
- **central controlling area** (medulla oblongata);
- **afferent neurones** (relaying information from receptors to the medulla);
- **efferent neurones** (transmitting signals from the medulla to effector organs).

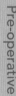

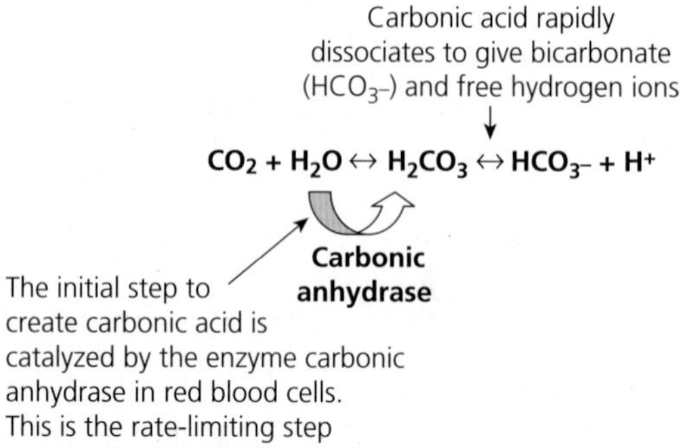

Carbonic acid rapidly
dissociates to give bicarbonate
(HCO_3-) and free hydrogen ions
↓

$$CO_2 + H_2O \leftrightarrow H_2CO_3 \leftrightarrow HCO_3- + H^+$$

**Carbonic
anhydrase**

The initial step to
create carbonic acid is
catalyzed by the enzyme carbonic
anhydrase in red blood cells.
This is the rate-limiting step

Fig. 1.6 Bicarbonate formation.

MICRO-facts

Bicarbonate ions are pumped out of red blood cells (RBCs) via chloride shift (which is a description of the replacement of bicarbonate ions with chloride ions to maintain electroneutrality of the RBC). The presence of carbonic anhydrase causes the rise in H^+ concentration in response to increased CO_2. The H^+ concentration in venous and tissue capillaries is higher than in arterial blood and it increases with increasing metabolic activity, reducing the pH.

Medulla oblongata

- The medulla contains the respiratory centre:
  - An automatic pattern of breathing is initiated by the medulla via:
    - inspiratory neurones (active only during inspiration);
    - expiratory neurones (active only during expiration).
  - This pattern is entirely automatic, but can be modulated by information from afferent receptors.

Afferent neurones

- The afferent limb of respiratory control consists of many different receptors picking up chemical signs of an increased requirement for O_2, or a build-up of CO_2.
- The receptors able to convey this are:
  - **chemoreceptors**, located:
    - **centrally** in the fourth ventricle;
    - **peripherally** in the carotid and aortic bodies (groups of chemoreceptors near the bifurcation of the common carotids and the aortic arch respectively).
  - There are also other receptors in the brain and lung.

MICRO-facts

- Opioids reduce the effect of an increased CO_2 on respiratory drive and therefore cause respiratory depression.
- Inhaled volatile anaesthetics can do this, to a lesser degree. They also modulate pulmonary blood flow, which compounds the V/Q mismatch of anaesthesia.

Central chemoreceptors

- These scan the pH of cerebrospinal fluid (CSF) in the ventricles (pH > 7.4 shows alkaline conditions caused by a decrease in H^+; pH < 7.4 shows acidic conditions caused by an increase in H^+):
  - Acidity requires more CO_2 to be eliminated and therefore these receptors stimulate an increased breathing rate (e.g. in diabetic ketoacidosis).
  - Low CO_2 levels and relatively alkaline CSF will do the opposite and cause a decrease in respiration to allow more CO_2 to accumulate.

MICRO-facts

A low CO_2 during external ventilation during anaesthesia can precipitate delayed spontaneous ventilation via this mechanism.

Peripheral chemoreceptors

- These monitor the partial pressure of O_2 and CO_2 in the blood and stimulate increased breathing rate if the partial pressure of O_2 is <10 kPa or the CO_2 is >5 kPa:
  - The carotid body relays information to the respiration centre via the **glossopharyngeal nerve** (cranial nerve (CN) IX) and the aortic body does so via the **vagus nerve** (CN X).
  - These receptors are thought to be the quickest mechanism to modulate the respiratory rate.

Lungs

- These receptors carry out several functions, but are all carried to the medulla via the vagus nerve:
  - Receptors in the walls of the bronchi detect substances that may cause damage or irritate the lungs and initiate a cough or sneeze reflex.
  - Receptors in elastic tissues (in both the lungs and chest wall) respond to stretching of the lungs and avoid inspiration if the lungs are already stretched. This avoids overdistension and lung damage.
  - Receptors in pulmonary blood vessels stimulate the respiratory centre when vessels are stretched, which can occur in heart failure.

Pre-operative

Other brain areas

Other areas of the brain are able to override central control of respiration to allow conscious control of breathing.

- There are several mechanisms which result in areas of the brain, other than the medulla, taking over control of respiration:
  - **strong emotional stimuli**: a traumatic experience can cause hyperventilation;
  - **prior to strenuous exercise**: deep ventilation may occur in preparation;
  - **massive haemorrhage**: hyperventilation is initiated by the autonomic nervous system at the hypothalamus and vasomotor control centre.

MICRO-facts

Remember the mnemonic: **C3, 4, 5 keeps your diaphragm alive!**

Efferent neurones

- Efferent supply from the medulla innervates:
  - the diaphragm (phrenic nerve, from spinal nerves C3, 4 and 5):
    - the diaphragm is the most important respiratory muscle. Damage to the spinal cord above C3 is usually fatal because of no respiratory effort;
  - intercostal muscles (intercostal nerves leaving the spine from T1 and 2);
  - accessory muscles: sternocleidomastoid, scalene muscles, trapezius, latisimus dorsi (supplied by nerves of the cervical plexus) and abdominal muscles, e.g. rectus abdominis.
- Inspiration is an active process and requires stimulation from the respiratory centre.
- Expiration is passive at normal respiration rates.

MICRO-reference

If more details about respiratory physiology are required, **Respiratory Physiology** by JB West (Baltimore, MD: Lippincott, Williams & Wilkins, 2008) is considered to be a very good source of information.

1.3 CARDIOVASCULAR PHYSIOLOGY

ELECTROPHYSIOLOGY OF THE HEART

The heart must be able to control two systems within one organ. Precision in the contraction of both atria and ventricles is necessary to ensure simultaneous contraction of both sides.

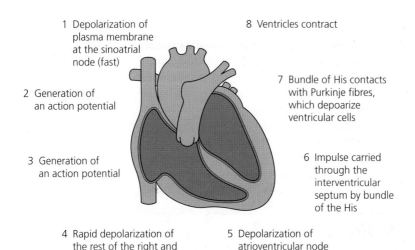

1 Depolarization of plasma membrane at the sinoatrial node (fast)

2 Generation of an action potential

3 Generation of an action potential

4 Rapid depolarization of the rest of the right and left atrium

5 Depolarization of atrioventricular node (slow) and atrial contraction

6 Impulse carried through the interventricular septum by bundle of the His

7 Bundle of His contacts with Purkinje fibres, which depoarize ventricular cells

8 Ventricles contract

Fig. 1.7 **Sequence of events in the cardiac cycle.**

Impulse initiation

- This is by depolarization of the plasma membrane:
  - Cardiac muscle differs from skeletal muscle in that an impulse can be generated with no external excitation: **cardiac muscle automaticity**.
  - Most muscle cells have an action potential induced by a motor neurone; the initial depolarization is caused by Na^+ influx, which triggers Ca^{2+} release from the sarcoplasmic reticulum.
  - Ca^{2+} release from the sarcoplasmic reticulum is induced by an influx of Ca^{2+} via voltage-gated calcium channels. This is different from skeletal muscle, where it is generated by depolarization, and is a mechanism to increase the total Ca^{2+}: **calcium-induced calcium release**.
- Repolarization occurs by K^+ release from cells.
- However, different myocardial cells are able to depolarize at different rates, such as the sinoatrial (SA) region, as a result of the increased number of f-channels (more details below) and therefore pass on action potentials at different rates; this is vital for the heart to contract effectively.

MICRO-facts

Myocardial cells are able to conduct impulses well because each cell is joined to another by an intercalated disc. Gap junctions adjacent to the intercalated discs provide a conduction system for the impulse generated at the sinoatrial node.

Excitation–contraction coupling

- The process by which the initiation of an action potential and the contraction of cardiac muscle are synchronized.
- It occurs as a result of an increased intra-cellular Ca^{2+} concentration:
  - This cytosolic calcium is able to bind to troponin. This exposes the actin-binding sites so actin–myosin bridges can form.
  - This results in contraction of the fibre and therefore contraction of the whole muscle segment.

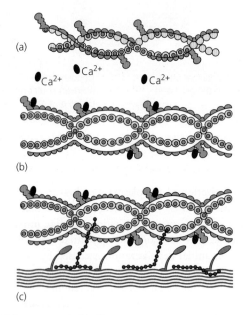

Fig. 1.8 (a–c) Calcium–troponin binding.

CARDIAC CYCLE

The cardiac cycle is split into systole and diastole.

Diastole

- Early diastole:
  - ventricular relaxation means that the pressure is low, allowing the majority of filling to occur;
  - repolarization also occurs during this phase.
- Mid- to late diastole:
  - the atria and ventricles are both relaxed;
  - the ventricular pressure rises (as blood flows in);

- the SA node discharges and the atrium depolarizes;
- the atria contract synchronously (known as **atrial kick**), filling the ventricles with an extra 20–30% of blood, to reach the end-diastolic volume (**EDV**) within the ventricles.

Systole

- The impulse reaches the atrioventricular (AV) node and is conducted via the bundle of His and Purkinje fibres, leading to ventricular muscle contraction.
- Contraction causes a sharp increase in ventricular pressure, so immediately closes the AV valves, preventing backflow to the atria.
- There is a brief period during which the rising pressure in the ventricles still does not exceed that in the aorta – isovolumetric contraction.
- When the pressure is high enough, the aortic and pulmonary valves open and blood is ejected via isotonic contraction.
- There is a lower pressure in the pulmonary system owing to the large alveolar surface and thin vasculature aiding gas exchange; this explains the less muscular right ventricle.
- The **stroke volumes** (the volume of blood ejected from one ventricle in each heart beat) from the left and right ventricles are the same:
  - stroke volume (SV) = EDV (pre-load) − end-systolic volume (ESV);

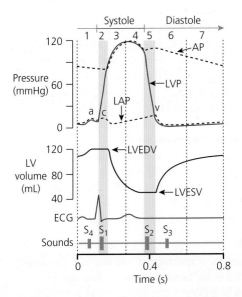

Fig. 1.9 The cardiac cycle. A, c, v (these are waveforms of the jugular venous pressure (JVP) or left atrial pressure (LAP)); AP, aortic pressure; LV, left ventricle; LVEDV, left ventricular end-diastolic volume; LVESV, left ventricular end-systolic volume; LVP, left ventricular pressure.

- some blood always remains in the ventricle after contraction and this volume is known as the ESV;
- typical volumes: SV, 70 mL; EDV, 135 mL; ESV, 65 mL.

Cardiac output

The volume of blood ejected from each ventricle per beat is more commonly combined and expressed as the volume per minute (in litres).
- **Cardiac output = Heart rate (HR) × SV.**
- Under normal circumstances the complete volume of blood is circulated round the body in 1 minute.

Heart rate

- The HR can be maintained in the absence of any external influence, owing to the autonomous firing at the SA node. The natural HR with no nervous interference would be around 100 beats/min.
- HR can be modified by:
  - **Parasympathetic** action (vagus nerve):
    - Causes a decrease in HR.
    - **Neurotransmitter**: acetylcholine.
    - **Receptors**: muscarinic.
    - Parasympathetic control prevails at rest decreasing the natural HR to around 70 beats/min.
    - The influx of Na^+ into the cells is reduced, causing the threshold plasma membrane potential to be reached more slowly. In addition, parasympathetic innervation hyperpolarizes the cell membranes by increasing permeability to K^+.
  - **Sympathetic** action:
    - Causes increased HR.
    - **Neurotransmitter**: adrenaline.
    - **Receptor**: β-adrenergic.
    - This is achieved by increasing the influx of Na^+ via f-type channels, allowing the threshold plasma potential to be reached more quickly and action potentials to be fired more rapidly.
  - Other factors:
    - Temperature, pH, adenosine, some hormones.

Stroke volume

- Increased strength of contraction will increase the stroke volume.
- There are three main factors that will affect the SV:
  - changes in EDV;
  - changes in sympathetic stimulation of the ventricles;
  - changes in the afterload, such as arterial pressure (increased with artery stenosis or atheromatous vessels).

- The Frank–Starling mechanism explains the relationship between SV and EDV:
  - The greater the EDV, the greater the SV. This is because the bigger the EDV, the more stretched each muscle fibre will be. This will result in a larger contraction and, therefore, a greater stroke volume and an increase in heart rate (the **Bainbridge reflex**).
  - The Frank–Starling curve shows the importance in this relationship, as increased venous return will automatically increase output. This prevents congestive build-up of blood.

Afterload

- This is the resistance to ventricular ejection of blood.
- Also known as peripheral vascular resistance (PVR):
  - This is determined by the diameter of vessels such as arterioles and capillaries and by pre-capillary sphincters.

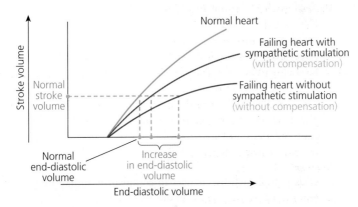

Fig. 1.10 Frank–Starling curve.

  - Narrower vessels increase the PVR and therefore increase afterload, which in turn reduces SV and HR (a **baroreceptor reflex**).

SYSTEMIC CIRCULATION

The systemic circulation describes the arteries, arterioles, capillaries and veins, which perfuse all tissues within the body.

Blood pressure

Arterial BP is reliant on compliance of vessels and blood volume.
- **Systolic BP (SBP):**
  - The maximum arterial pressure during ventricular ejection.

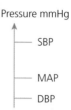

Fig. 1.11 Systolic (SBP), diastolic (DBP) and mean (MAP) blood pressures.

- **Diastolic BP (DBP)**:
  - Minimum arterial pressure, occurring just before blood is ejected from the ventricles.
- **Pulse pressure (PP)**:
  - This is the difference between the SBP and the DBP. It is felt when palpating an artery.
  - PP is affected by several variables:
    - SV;
    - speed of SV ejection;
    - arterial compliance (which reduces with age and arteriosclerosis).
- **Mean arterial pressure (MAP)**:
  - The most accurate reflection of how well a person is maintaining perfusion is their MAP.
  - MAP cannot be derived by the average value between SBP and DBP, as diastole lasts longer than systole:

  $$MAP = DBP + 1/3(SBP - DBP)$$

  - MAP is not affected by changes in compliance, unlike PP.
  - It denotes the average of the entire cardiac cycle.

Control of blood pressure

There are many factors which influence systemic BP.

- **Neurone-independent control of systemic BP**:
  - Active hyperaemia:
    - This is increased blood flow as a result of increased metabolic activity.
    - The increased blood flow is caused by arteriolar vasodilatation.
    - Factors which induce active hyperaemia:
      - $\uparrow CO_2$;
      - $\downarrow pH$ ($\uparrow$ free H^+);
      - breakdown products of ATP;
      - K^+, from repeated action potentials;
      - breakdown products of membrane phospholipids;

  ○ bradykinin;
  ○ nitric oxide.
- Reactive hyperaemia:
  - This is the process which occurs as blood flow is restored to a tissue after vascular occlusion:
    ○ vasodilatation occurs (owing to the factors which induce hyperaemia discussed above);
    ○ when blood is able to get back to the vessels, they have a much wider diameter, causing a large increase in flow.
- Flow autoregulation:
  - a change in blood pressure can alter tissue perfusion;
  - a further change in arteriolar resistance (by vasodilatation or vasoconstriction) is able to alter flow and therefore ensure adequate perfusion;
  - this is known as autoregulation.
- Injury:
  - tissue injury causes vasoconstriction, mediated by substances released directly from the damaged tissue.
- Hormones:
  - Adrenaline (from the renal medulla):
    ○ able to bind α-adrenergic receptors on arteriolar smooth muscle;
    ○ this causes vasoconstriction in high concentrations; however, in low concentrations it causes vasodilatation because of its β activity.
  - Angiotensin II (part of the renin–angiotensin system; see Chapter 10, Post-operative fluids): causes vasoconstriction.
  - Anti-diuretic hormone: causes some vasoconstriction.
  - Atrial naturietic peptide: causes some vasodilatation.
- **Nervous regulation of systemic BP**:
  - sympathetic neurones;
  - parasympathetic;
  - autonomic non-adrenergic, non-cholinergic;
  - baroreceptors;
  - central control.

CARDIOVASCULAR SYSTEM RESPONSE TO ANAESTHESIA

- Anaesthetic agents:
  - Cause a degree of cardiac depression, which reduces cardiac contractility.
  - Some also decrease sympathetic stimulation of the systemic system, which causes vasodilatation.

- The combined effect is to decrease blood pressure and therefore potentially compromise perfusion to the major organs, particularly at induction of anaesthesia.
- **Inhaled volatile agents** (see Chapter 7, Drugs in the anaesthetic room):
    - can decrease the rate of firing from the SA node, leading to the AV node taking over, creating 'junctional' rhythms (the ECG shows either no P waves or the P wave bears no relation to the QRS complex).

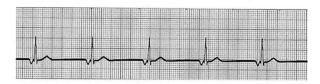

Fig. 1.12 Electrocardiogram: junctional/complete heart block.

- **Local anaesthetics (e.g. lidocaine)** (if given systemically):
    - depress conduction of cardiac impulses;
    - can cause cardiac arrest at high doses.
- **Spinal and epidural agents** (see Chapter 6, Local and regional anaesthesia):
    - These block sympathetic nerves as well as sensory and motor nerves.
    - This can lead to:
        - hypotension, as a result of arterial and venous dilation as peripheral nerves are blocked;
        - blockage of sympathetic fibres from the thoracic spine supplying the myocardium, which counteracts the parasympathetic control of the HR (from the vagus nerve) and causes bradycardia if the block is high enough. This prevents an appropriate increase in HR in response to hypotension.

1.4 NEUROPHYSIOLOGY

CELLS OF THE NERVOUS SYSTEM

Neurone

- **Function**:
    - generating and transmitting electrical signals from cell to cell;
    - this process commonly uses chemical messengers, named neurotransmitters.
- **Structure**:
    - **Processes**, which connect with other cells. There are three main types of process:
        - **Dendrites**:
            - ○ these extend from the cell body and contain many branches;

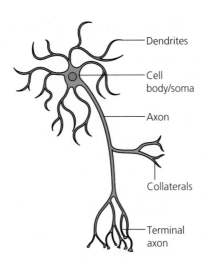

Fig. 1.13 A simple neurone.

- ○ receive most of the input from other neurones (along with the cell body).
  - **Axon**:
    - ○ also known as a nerve cell fibre;
    - ○ extend away from the cell body to carry the electrical impulse to neighbouring cells;
    - ○ can have branches, called collaterals;
    - ○ towards the end of the axon, they undergo further branching (increasing the potential to make contact with a greater number of cells and therefore spread the impulse more widely).
  - **Axon terminals**:
    - ○ The final part of the axon is characterized by many small branches from which neurotransmitters are released (see later in this chapter under Synapses).
    - ○ Some cells are able to release neurotransmitters at other points of the axon, known as varicosities.
- **Axon myelination**:
  - ● Myelin:
    - – This is an important feature of neurones, as it allows smooth, rapid electrical transmission to occur.
    - – Formed by oligodendrocytes in the central nervous system (CNS) and Schwann cells in the peripheral nervous system.
    - – Made up of lipid and protein, forming a modified plasma membrane.
- **Classes of neurones**:
  - ● **Efferent**: (1) These relay signals from the CNS to effector organs; the cell bodies reside in the CNS, with the axons extending peripherally.

(2) Bundles of efferent and afferent neurones create the nerves of the peripheral nervous system.
- **Afferent**: (1) These relay information from the organs and tissues via sensory receptors to the CNS. (2) These cells are slightly different from most other neurones; they have a long single process (or axon) with a cell body positioned along the length of the axon. (3) One end of the axon synapses with peripheral receptors, bringing the signal in. The other synapses with other neurones and enters the CNS.
- **Interneurones**: (1) These reside in the CNS and make up around 99% of all neurones. (2) They serve many different functions, such as changing the type of signal relayed or blocking a signal. (3) They are an integral part of many nerve transmissions.

ELECTRICAL PROPAGATION

Several factors are involved in the generation of an electrical current.

Cellular compartment compositions
- Extra-cellular fluid:
  - main solutes are sodium and chloride (Na^+ and Cl^-).
- Intra-cellular fluid:
  - mainly potassium (K^+) and particles that have a charge but are unable to diffuse (e.g. proteins with charged side chains or phosphate compounds).

Potential difference
- The different compositions of ionic compounds in the intra- and extra-cellular fluids cause a difference in overall charge that is maintained by Na/K-ATPase pumps (active transport).
- The separation of charges (by a cell membrane) produces a potential difference (measured in millivolts), also known more simply as a potential.
- This difference in charge or potential promotes movement, which creates a current.

MICRO-facts

Ohm's law

This states that the movement of electricity (current) through a substance is affected by the magnitude of potential difference and resistance:

$$I = V/R$$

where I is current, V is voltage and R is resistance.

Current

- Current will be affected by:
  - A large **potential difference** in charge, which will create a faster flow.
  - **Resistance** to flow, which can be created by the substance in which the current must move:
    - conductors and ion channels in membrane: these facilitate faster flow (such as water with dissolved ions);
    - insulators: these lead to very slow flow (such as lipid membranes).

Resting membrane potential

- This is the potential difference between the inside and outside of the cell.
- The inside is generally negative in relation to the outside because of the Na/K-ATPase channels.
- This means that:
  - due to attraction, some of the negative ions inside the cell line the membrane and some of the extra-cellular positive ions line the outside of the membrane;
  - this creates a charged shell around the cell.
- The value of the resting membrane potential is deduced by assigning the extra-cellular compartment zero. This allows the membrane potential to be valued according to the magnitude of negative intra-cellular charge:
  - If the difference in charge across the membrane is 45 mV, the membrane potential would be 45 mV; this varies between cells.
    - Neurones generally have a resting potential of between -40 and -90 mV.
  - The size of the membrane potential depends on:
    - the difference between the intra- and extra-cellular ion concentration (maintained by Na/K-ATPase);
    - differences in ion permeability.
- A resting membrane potential occurs by movement of ions, which happens for several reasons. Commonly:
  - **Concentration gradients**:
    - Ions will diffuse across to the other side if channels are open.
  - **Electrical potentials**:
    - Movement of ions by diffusion can change the charge on either side of the membrane, causing a change in membrane potential.
    - Ions can move back across the membrane, attracted by charge rather than by concentration.
    - When the movement of ions caused by concentration and electrical charge are equal, the **equilibrium potential** is reached.
  - The resting potential is achieved by the movement of K^+ out of the cell through open channels:

- The potential will not reach that of K^+, however, as Na^+ ions are also constantly diffusing into the cell.
- There are three main steps to create a resting potential:
  - Na^+ moves out and K^+ moves via Na/K-ATPase pumps.
  - The net movement of K^+ via K^+ channels exceeds the movement of Na^+ because the resting membrane is more permeable to K^+ than Na^+.
  - This movement balances out to create a stable resting potential.

MICRO-facts

- **Polarize**: there is a difference in charge between extra-cellular and intra-cellular compartments.
- **Repolarize**: return to a polarized state from a change in charge.
- **Hyperpolarize**: when the potential is more negative in relation to the resting potential value.
- **Depolarize**: the potential becomes less negative in relation to the resting potential.

Action potentials

- An action potential results from large changes in membrane potential.
- This change is very rapid and the membrane soon repolarizes back to resting potential.
- Muscles and some endocrine and immune cells are able to generate action potentials, along with neurones.
- There are certain properties which allow a membrane to generate an action potential. One important factor is the presence of voltage-gated channels:
  - **Voltage-gated channels**:
    - These channels open rapidly in response to depolarization of the membrane and inactivate once the membrane repolarizes.
    - Na^+ and K^+ voltage-gated channels allow an action potential to be generated. Na^+ channels tend to open first.
  - Sequence of events: see Fig. 1.15.
- **Refractory period**: this is the stage when an action potential cannot be generated:
  - **Absolute refractory periods** occur when an action potential is already occurring. A second stimulus will not generate another action potential as that section of membrane already contains open or inactivated Na^+ channels.

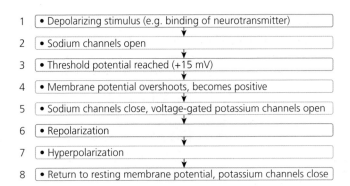

1 • Depolarizing stimulus (e.g. binding of neurotransmitter)

2 • Sodium channels open

3 • Threshold potential reached (+15 mV)

4 • Membrane potential overshoots, becomes positive

5 • Sodium channels close, voltage-gated potassium channels open

6 • Repolarization

7 • Hyperpolarization

8 • Return to resting membrane potential, potassium channels close

Fig. 1.14 Sequence of events in an action potential.

- **Relative refractory periods** occur after the absolute refractory period. It is possible to generate an action potential, but only if the stimulus is greater than that usually required to overcome the threshold potential.

SYNAPSES

Function

- Allows a neurone to pass a signal (chemical or electrical) to another cell.

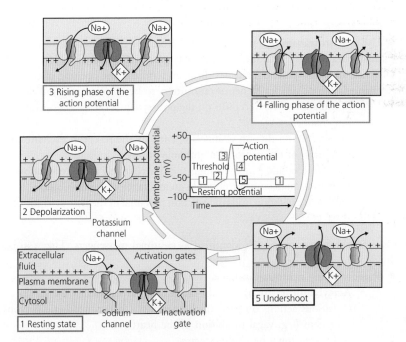

Fig. 1.15 Action potential generation.

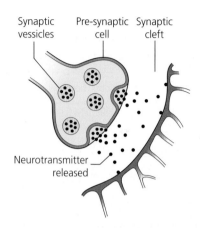

Fig. 1.16 A synapse.

Types of synapse

Electrical synapses

- Conduct electricity from one cell to another via open fluid channels such as gap junctions that allow ions to move freely between adjacent cells.
- Are used between visceral smooth muscle cells and cardiac muscle cells.

Chemical synapses

- Use a **neurotransmitter** to pass a signal from the **pre-synaptic** to the **post-synaptic** cell. The message can only pass in this direction.
- When an action potential reaches the axon terminal, the opening of calcium channels causes vesicles of neurotransmitters to be emptied into the cleft:
  - Stimulation of the receptors on the post-synaptic cell causes opening of ion channels.
  - Depending on the ion channels opened by the receptor, excitation or inhibition of the neuronal membrane occurs.
  - Increasing conductance through sodium channels causes excitation.
  - Increasing potassium or chloride conductance causes inhibition.
  - Sufficient excitation leads to an action potential in the post-synaptic cell.

Neurotransmitters

Over 50 substances have been identified as neuronal messengers. They can be divided by chemical class.

- Rapidly acting neurotransmitters:
  - **Acetylcholine (ACh)**: mostly excitatory (particularly in the CNS):
    - various actions on parts of the peripheral parasympathetic nervous system (e.g. vagal inhibition of the heart);
    - broken down by cholinesterase.

- Amines:
  - **Noradrenaline**: mainly excitatory:
    - ○ various actions on peripheral sympathetic nervous system (e.g. inhibition of the gastrointestinal (GI) tract).
  - **Adrenaline**: mainly excitatory:
    - ○ inhibitory in parts of the peripheral sympathetic nervous system (e.g. in the GI tract).
  - **Dopamine**: mainly inhibitory.
  - **Serotonin (5-hydroxytryptamine)**: mainly inhibitory:
    - ○ Inhibitor of pain pathways in the spinal cord and higher brain function related to mood and sleep.
  - **Histamine**.
- Amino acids:
  - **γ-aminobutyric acid**: always inhibitory.
  - **Glycine**: always inhibitory.
  - **Glutamate**: always excitatory.
  - **Aspartate**.
- **Nitric oxide**:
  - Works very differently from other neurotransmitters. It is synthesized when required and, rather than acting on the membrane, alters intra-cellular metabolism to modify excitability.
- Slowly acting transmitters, neuropeptides and growth factors:
  - are synthesized differently and act differently and more slowly (from hours to perhaps years) than the short-acting transmitters;
  - include hypothalamic releasing hormones, pituitary peptides (e.g. **adrenocorticotropic hormone**) and various other **growth factors** and **peptides**.

ORGANIZATION OF THE NERVOUS SYSTEM

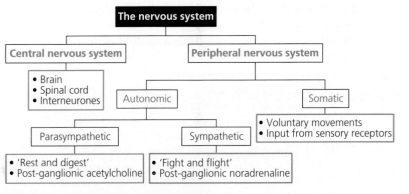

Fig. 1.17 Organization of the nervous system.

THE AUTONOMIC NERVOUS SYSTEM

Function

- Controls visceral functions in order to maintain homeostasis in the face of different physiological stressors:
  - acts by directly controlling or modulating function of various organs;
  - can act very rapidly (within seconds) to alter physiological parameters (such as heart rate and blood pressure);
  - controlled by centres in the **hypothalamus**, **brainstem** and **spinal cord**, which receive subconscious signals from visceral organs and respond with appropriate reflex signals to control the organ. Signals are sent via two neurones: the pre-ganglionic and post-ganglionic.
- Fibres are:
  - cholinergic (secreting acetylcholine); or
  - adrenergic (secreting noradrenaline).

Sympathetic nervous system

- Division of the nervous system responsible for the 'fight or flight' response; generally involved in preparing the body for periods of physiological stress.
- **Neuronal pathway**:
  - The pre-ganglionic cell body lies in the intermediolateral horn of the spinal cord.
  - Fibres pass into the ganglia of the sympathetic chain via the anterior root of the spinal cord, the spinal nerve and the white ramus.
  - The fibres then synapse with the post-ganglionic neurone at one of three places:
    - the ganglion at the level it leaves the spinal cord;
    - the ganglion above or below the level it leaves the spinal cord;
    - a peripheral sympathetic ganglion.
  - The location of the post-ganglionic neurone depends on the course of the pre-ganglionic fibre (which is in either the chain ganglion or a peripheral sympathetic ganglion).
  - The fibres from the post-ganglionic neurone then extend to the target organ.
  - Segmental distribution (approximation):
    - T1: fibres supply the head;
    - T2: fibres supply the neck;
    - T3–6: fibres supply the thorax;
    - T7–11: fibres supply the abdomen;
    - T11–L2: fibres supply the legs.

Transmitters and receptors

- The pre-ganglionic neurones of the sympathetic system are **cholinergic**.
- Post-ganglionic neurones are stimulated by ACh binding to nicotinic acetylcholine receptors (nAChRs) located on the post-synaptic neural membrane.
- The majority of post-ganglionic neurones of the sympathetic system are **adrenergic**. A minority, supplying sweat glands, piloerector muscles and a small number of blood vessels, secrete ACh:
    - There are two main types of adrenergic receptors:
        - Alpha (α).
        - Beta (β).
        - Noradrenaline excites α more then β, whereas adrenaline is an agonist for both. Each receptor group can be further divided into subgroups, the locations and functions of which are summarized in Table 1.1 and Table 1.2.

Table 1.1 Autonomic nervous system receptors, their locations and main effects.

Adrenergic receptors	LOCATIONS	MAIN EFFECTS
α_1	Blood vessel smooth muscle	Vasoconstriction
	GI tract smooth muscle	Intestinal relaxation
	Cardiac muscle	Weak positive inotrope
	Detrusor muscle	Mild detrusor contraction
	Pupil dilatory muscle	Pupil dilatation
α_2	Arteries	Vasodilatation
	Cardiac vessels	Vasoconstriction
	Veins	Vasoconstriction
	GI sphincters	Intestinal sphincter contraction
	Bladder sphincter	Bladder sphincter constriction
β_1	Heart muscle	Positive inotrope
		Positive chronotrope
	Juxtaglomerular cells	Renin secretion
β_2	Blood vessels	Vasodilatation
	Bronchioles	Bronchodilatation
	Liver	Gluconeogenesis
		Glycogenolysis
	Intestine	Intestinal relaxation
	Bladder wall	Bladder wall relaxation
	Uterus	Uterus relaxation
	Cardiac muscle	Weak positive ionotrope
		Weak positive chronotrope

Physiology

Table 1.2

Dopamine receptors	LOCATIONS	MAIN EFFECTS
D1, D2	Renal	Diuresis
D1, D4, D5	Cardiac	Increases cardiac contractility and cardiac output

Paraympathetic nervous system
- **Neuronal pathway**:
    - Parasympathetic fibres leave from CNs III, VII, IX, and X, and S1–4.
    - Roughly three-quarters of parasympathetic fibres are part of the vagus nerve (CN X).
    - The pre-ganglionic neurones pass all the way to the target organ.
    - Pre-ganglionic fibres synapse with post-ganglionic neurones located in the wall of the organ.
- **Nervous distribution**:
    - **CN III**: supplies the eye ciliary ganglion, ciliary muscles of the eye, papillary sphincter.
    - **CN VII**: supplies the lacrimal glands, submandibular and sublingual glands.
    - **CN IX**: supplies the otic ganglion and parotid gland.

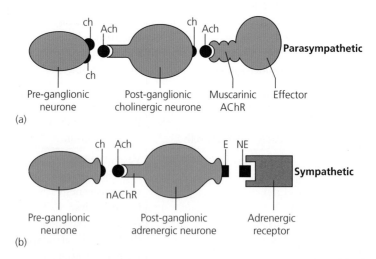

Fig. 1.18 (a and b) Transmitters and receptors. ACh, acetylcholine; AChR, acetylcholine receptor; nAChR, nicotinic acetylcholine receptor; E, adrenaline; NE, noradrenaline.

- **CN X**: supplies the heart, bronchi and lungs, stomach and parts of the small and large bowel.
- **S1–4**: supplies large bowel and urinary bladder.
- **Transmitters and receptors**:
  - The pre-ganglionic neurones of the parasympathetic system are **cholinergic.**
  - Post-ganglionic neurones are stimulated by ACh binding to nAChRs located on the post-synaptic neural membrane.
  - The majority of post-ganglionic neurones of the parasympathetic system are cholinergic.
  - ACh stimulates muscarinic acetylcholine receptors on the target organ to exert its effect.

2 Preparing for surgery

2.1 BASIC PRINCIPLES OF ANAESTHESIA

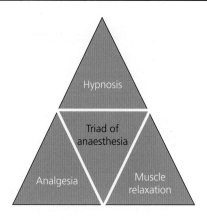

Fig. 2.1 Triad of anaesthesia.

- **Triad of anaesthesia**: the fundamental principles behind anaesthesia consist of three strands:
    - **hypnosis**: an altered state of consciousness;
    - **muscle relaxation**: paralysis of all voluntary muscles;
    - **analgesia**: the relief of pain.
- **Sedation**: induced, reversible reduction in conscious level, to a level where the patient should be rousable to voice or light touch.

2.2 PRE-OPERATIVE ASSESSMENT

AIMS OF PRE-OPERATIVE ASSESSMENT

Thorough pre-operative assessment has been proven to improve outcome and reduce post-operative length of stay. Every patient must be assessed prior to the administration of anaesthesia for several reasons:

- to ascertain the most appropriate anaesthetic technique to use;
- to explain the anaesthetic technique to the patient;
- to identify underlying conditions that would increase the patient's peri-operative risk;
- to discuss pre-, peri- and post-operative risks with the patient;
- to reassure the patient;
- to obtain informed consent.

CLINICAL ASSESSMENT FOR ELECTIVE ADMISSION

Planned surgery/Procedure	Consultant	Patient I.D.

Base line observations at assessment.		Allergies/Reactions
B.P........../..............	Urinalysis...............	
Temp.........................	Peak flow...............	
Pulse.......................	Resp.....................	
Weight ....kg	BMI......................	
Height...............cm 0₂ SATS..................		Latex sensitivity

Medical History

Cardiovascular

1.	Myocardial infarction	NO	YES	....
2.	Angina	NO	YES	....
3.	Chest pain	NO	YES	....
4.	Hypertension	NO	YES	....
5.	Rheumatic fever	NO	YES	....
6.	Palpitations	NO	YES	....
7.	Pacemaker	NO	YES	....
8.	Faints	NO	YES	....
9.	Severe headaches	NO	YES	....
10.	Blackouts	NO	YES	....
11.	Dizzy spells	NO	YES	....
12.	Cerebrovascular accident	NO	YES	....
13.	Bilateral ankle swelling	NO	YES	....
14.	Previous thrombosis	NO	YES	....
15.	Exercise tolerance			....
16.	Anaemia / blood disorder /	NO	YES	....
	Bleed or bruise easily			....

Respiratory

17.	Asthma/Chronic airways disease	NO	YES	....
18.	Breathlessness/Wheeze	NO	YES	....
19.	Chest Infection/Cold	NO	YES	....
20.	Bronchitis/Emphysema	NO	YES	....
	Tuberculosis/Pneumonia	NO	YES	....
21.	Sleep apnoea	NO	YES	....
22.	Smoker	NO	YES	....

(Patient aware of the risk to health by smoking and given advice leaflet regarding stopping smoking. Informed of the Trust No Smoking Policy)

Fig. 2.2a Example of pre-anaesthesia assessment questionnaire.

Pre-operative

Gastro intestinal

23. Indigestion / hiatus hernia
    Ulcers / Gastritis　　　　　　　　NO　　　　　YES　　.........................

24. Colitis / P.R. blood
    Diarrhoea / Constipation　　　　　NO　　　　　YES　　.........................

25. Jaundice / Liver disease　　　　　NO　　　　　YES　　.........................

26. Diabetes　　　　　　　　　　　　NO　　　　　YES　　.........................

27. Special dietary needs..

28. Alcohol intake...................................... (units per day / week)

Genito-Urinary

29. Urinary problems　　　　　　　　NO　　　　　YES　　.........................

30. Kidney disease　　　　　　　　　NO　　　　　YES　　.........................

Functional

31. Muscular disease / weakness　　　　　　　　　　　　.........................
    Tingling / numbness　　　　　　　NO　　　　　YES　　.........................
    Specific illness:　　Myasthenia gravis - Motor neurone - Multiple sclerosis – Poliomyelitis

32. Eyesight / Hearing problems　　　　NO　　　　　YES　　.........................

33. Epilepsy / Fits　　　　　　　　　NO　　　　　YES　　.........................

34. Mobility　...
    ....

35. In the case of female patient, is their any possibility of pregnancy　NO / YES
    Date of LMP　...................................

    Patient advised to avoid becoming pregnant prior to admission for the proposed surgical procedure　☐

Other

36. Eczema　　　　　　　　　　　　NO　　　　　YES　　.........................

37. Skin lesions　　　　　　　　　　NO　　　　　YES　　.........................
    Area/s affected...

Previous surgery / illness	Anaesthetic history
	Inc previous intubation/anaesthetic problems / history of close family anaesthetic problems, eg. suxamethonium apnoea, malignant hyperthermia
....	....
....	....
....	....
....	....
....	....
....	....

Fig. 2.2b Pre-anaesthesia assessment questionnaire.

PRE-OPERATIVE ASSESSMENT CLINIC

- Where patients are assessed depends on:
  - the type of surgery planned (e.g. elective surgery or emergency procedure);
  - the patient's condition.
- Most assessment now takes place in specifically designed clinics:
  - assessment of patients ahead of the day of surgery is preferable to assessment immediately prior to surgery;

- many patients may then be admitted on the day of surgery;
- greater numbers of patients may be seen per surgical list;
- pre-operative baseline investigations, e.g. bloods, ECGs, may be done and problem results addressed prior to the day of surgery.

METHODS OF ASSESSMENT

Patients will usually be assessed by a specialist nurse. The assessment follows a set structure:

- **Pre-anaesthetic questionnaires** can be used as a preliminary screening tool, prior to assessment in a clinic.
- **History, examination and investigations** identify any factors which may affect the patient's safety while under anaesthesia.
- **Patients requiring emergency surgery** will often be assessed in the acute setting and this assessment will usually be integrated into the resuscitation and preparation of the patient for surgery.

2.3 ASSESSMENT OF SURGICAL RISK

THE AMERICAN SOCIETY OF ANESTHESIOLOGISTS (ASA) GRADING SYSTEM

- The health status of all patients in the UK is assessed prior to surgery.
- The ASA grade patients receive correlates with their peri-operative mortality:
  1) Normal healthy patient.
  2) Mild systemic disease, no functional limitation.
  3) Moderate systemic disease, with functional limitations.
  4) Severe systemic disease, which is a constant threat to life.
  5) Moribund patient unlikely to survive 24 hours with or without operation.
  6) Declared brain dead patient whose organs are being removed for donor purposes.

CARDIAC RISK SCORING

- Particular consideration should also be given to the patient's potential risk of myocardial infarction (MI), as this is the most common serious anaesthetic complication. The **Goldman cardiac risk index** (Tables 2.1 and 2.2) scoring system is used for patients with a history of cardiac disease, undergoing non-cardiac surgery.
- The score correlates with the risk of peri-operative MI.

Table 2.1 Goldman risk index: part 1

PATIENT FACTORS	POINTS
History	
Age >70 years	5
MI within 6 months	10
Examination	
Third heart sound, raised JVP	11
Significant aortic stenosis	3
ECG	
Non-sinus rhythm or presence of premature atrial complexes	7
>5 ventricular ectopics per minute	7
General condition	
PaO_2 <8 kPa or $PaCO_2$ >7.5 kPa on air	3
K^+ <3.0 mmol/L; HCO_3^- <20 mmol/L	3
Urea >8.5 mmol/L; creatinine >200 mmol/L	3
Chronic liver disease	3
Bedridden from non-cardiac cause	3
Operation	
Intraperitoneal, intrathoracic, aortic	3
Emergency surgery	4

JVP, jugular venous pressure; MI, myocardial infarction.
Source: Gwinnutt CL. *Lecture notes: clinical anaesthesia*. Oxford, UK: Wiley-Blackwell, 2004.

Table 2.2 Goldman risk index: part 2

POINTS	RISK OF MI
Class I 0–5	1%
Class II 6–12	5%
Class III 13–25	16%
Class IV >26	56%

Source: Gwinnutt CL. *Lecture notes: clinical anaesthesia*. Oxford, UK: Wiley-Blackwell, 2004.

- Another way to assess a patient's ability to withstand the insult of major surgery is a form of exercise tolerance testing.
- One such system is **cardiopulmonary exercise testing**, which provides analysis of respiratory gas exchange and cardiac function at rest and during exercise.

2.4 ASSESSMENT OF AIRWAYS

The airway assessment is a vitally important part of the pre-operative assessment, as an unanticipated difficult intubation could prove fatal.

CLINICAL ASSESSMENT OF THE AIRWAY

Methods of clinical assessment of the airway include:

- **Inspection** of the patient's anatomy:
    - any limitation in mouth opening;
    - teeth (number, positioning and decay);
    - tongue (size);
    - swelling of soft tissue;
    - tracheal or laryngeal deviation;
    - any stiffness in the cervical spine.
- **Modified Mallampati technique** (MMT):
    - MMT requires the patient to sit opposite the anaesthetist, with their mouth wide open and tongue protruding.
    - This should allow a full view of the structures at the back of the patient's mouth.
    - **Grading system:**
        - **Class I**: faucial pillars, soft palate and uvula visible.
        - **Class II**: faucial pillars and soft palate visible. Uvula hidden by the base of the tongue.
        - **Class III**: only hard and soft palate visible.
        - **Class IV**: only hard palate visible.

MICRO-facts

A useful mnemonic for the risk factors for difficult intubation:

Overweight (BMI > 26)

Bearded

Elderly (> 55 years)

Snorers

Endentulous (without a full set of teeth)

Think of Father Christmas!

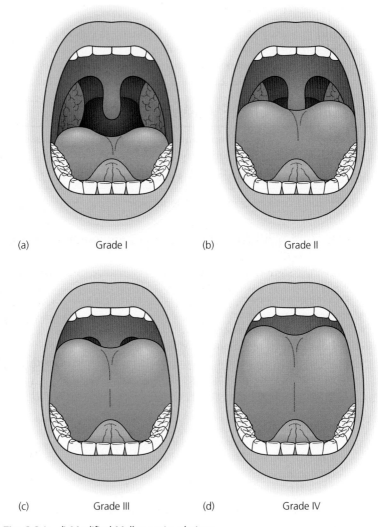

(a)   Grade I   (b)   Grade II

(c)   Grade III   (d)   Grade IV

Fig. 2.3 (a–d) Modified Mallampati technique.

INDICATORS FOR DIFFICULT INTUBATION

- **Wilson risk factors**:
  - Give the patient a score out of 10 according to their risk.
  - The factors scored are:
    - obesity;
    - restricted head and neck movements;
    - restricted jaw movements;

- receding mandible;
- protruding teeth.
- A score of >2 will predict approximately 75% of all difficult intubations.

2.5 INVESTIGATIONS TO CONSIDER

Investigations should only be requested when appropriate for the patient, considering their health, age and the type of operation.

- **Blood tests**:
  - **Full blood count**: to screen for anaemia and infection.
  - **Urea and electrolytes**: to screen for possible electrolyte disturbances or renal impairment.
  - **Liver function tests**: indications would be known hepatic disease, metastatic disease or malnutrition.
  - **Clotting screen/international normalized ratio (INR)**: to assess for bleeding risk.
  - **Crossmatch/group and save**: indicated for surgery when significant blood loss may occur, to ensure availability of blood products.
  - **Glucose/haemoglobin A_{1c}**: indicated for patients with diabetes, severe peripheral arterial disease or those taking long-term steroids to assess glucose control.
  - **Other tests for known diagnoses**:
    - **Haematinics/iron studies**: to investigate the cause of anaemia.
    - **Sickle cell screen**: patients with a family history of sickle cell disease.
    - **Thyroid function**: patients with a history of thyroid disease.
- **Urinalysis**:
  - to screen for urinary tract infections and abnormalities.
- **Lung function tests**:
  - **Spirometry**:
    - in patients with severe dyspnoea on mild to moderate exertion.
  - **Arterial blood gases**:
    - in patients dyspnoeic at rest or due for thoracic surgery.
- **Chest radiograph**:
  - indications include thoracic surgery, cardiac/respiratory disease, known or suspected malignancy or those from a region with endemic tuberculosis.
- **Electrocardiograph (ECG)**:
  - indications include hypertension, possible ischaemic heart disease (IHD), arrhythmia, diabetes mellitus.
- **Echocardiography**:
  - used to assess left ventricular function in patients with IHD or valvular disease.

Pre-operative

2.6 PRE-OPERATIVE MEDICATIONS

The 'Six As'. Pre-medications refer to drugs given before and in addition to those used for the induction (Table 2.3).

Patients were once universally pre-medicated, usually with morphine to sedate them. Pre-medication is now reserved for patients with concurrent medical illness, those who are particularly anxious or those who are at risk of anaesthetic-induced problems.

Table 2.3 Pre-operative medications

CATEGORY	DRUGS USED		REASON FOR USE
	CLASS	EXAMPLE	
Anxiolysis	Benzodiazepine	Temazepam Diazepam Lorazepam	Well absorbed Provide mild sedation and amnesia
	β-blocker	Atenolol	Anxiety
Amnesia	Benzodiazepine	Lorazepam	Provide anterograde amnesia
Anti-emetic	Dopamine (D$_2$) antagonist	Metoclopramide Domperidone Prochlorperazine	Increases gastric emptying Opiate and post-operative induced nausea
	Anti-histamines	Cyclizine	Post-operative induced nausea
	5HT$_3$ antagonists	Ondansetron	Severe/resistant nausea and vomiting
Antacid	H$_2$ antagonist Proton pump inhibitor	Ranitidine Omeprazole	To reduce risk of regurgitation/ aspiration at induction
Anti-autonomic	Anti-cholinergic Anti-sympathomimetic	Glycopyrrolate β-blocker	Reduce salivation
Analgesia	Opiates/opioids	Morphine Fentanyl	Sedation and analgesia

Pre-operative

2.7 MANAGEMENT OF REGULAR MEDICATIONS

DRUGS TO CONSIDER BEFORE SURGERY

- Various medications that a patient may be taking can complicate the anaesthetist's job, and must be considered (Table 2.4).

Table 2.4 Drugs to consider before surgery.

DRUG	EFFECT
Anti-coagulants	Increase peri-operative bleeding Haematoma at spinal/epidural site Complicate traumatic intubation
β-blockers	Bradycardia (but shown to be cardioprotective)
Calcium channel antagonists	Bradyarrhythmias
Contraceptive pill	Increase risk of thromboembolism
Digoxin	Arrhythmias Decreased cardiac output
Diuretics	Hypovolaemia (and unstable blood pressure), hypokalaemia and arrhythmias
Insulin	Hypoglycaemia
Monoamine oxidase inhibitors	Interact with some opioids Hypertensive response to vasoconstrictive agents
P450 inducers (e.g. anti-convulsants)	May increase requirement of anaesthetic/sedative agents.
Steroids	Adrenal suppression

DRUGS TO STOP BEFORE SURGERY

- Although most drug regimes remain unchanged prior to surgery, it is advised to stop some, including angiotensin-converting enzyme (ACE) inhibitors and angiotensin II receptor agonists following reports of dangerous hypotension during induction.
- Important drugs which must be stopped or increased prior to surgery are shown in Table 2.5.

Pre-operative

Table 2.5 Drugs to stop or increase before surgery

DRUG	REDUCE/STOP	INCREASE/CONTINUE
Warfarin	Should be stopped at least 3 days pre-operatively and the INR should be <1.5 (lower if regional techniques are to be used). Full anti-coagulation is an absolute contraindication for spinal/epidural	
Aspirin/clopidogrel	Should be stopped 7–14 days pre-operatively	
NSAIDs	Stopped at least 3 days pre-operatively in some centres	
ACE inhibitors and angiotensin II receptor antagonists	Stop 24 hours pre-operatively if taking for hypertension and blood pressure generally well controlled	
Oral contraceptives	Combined oral contraceptives should be stopped at least 4 weeks pre-operatively	Progesterone only pills can be continued
Steroids		Regular steroids should be increased during surgery. If patient NBM, intravenous steroids should be given

ACE, angiotensin-converting enzyme; INR, international normalized ratio; NBM, nil by mouth; NSAID, non-steroidal anti-inflammatory drug.

WARFARIN BRIDGING PROTOCOLS

- Warfarin is a long-acting and unpredictable anti-coagulant; in comparison, low molecular weight heparin (LMWH), e.g. enoxaparin, is shorter acting and more predictable.
- Bridging protocols involve stopping warfarin and replacing its actions with enoxaparin.

- Bridging protocols generally follow this sequence:
  - warfarin stopped around 5 days prior to surgery;
  - INR checked and enoxaparin started the day prior to surgery;
  - warfarin restarted after surgery alongside enoxaparin;
  - LMWH stopped after the INR is in therapeutic range for two consecutive days;
  - bridging protocols also exist for intravenous heparin, which may be used when tighter and more immediate control is required. These protocols require regular blood tests for activated partial thromboplastin time and the intravenous infusion must be monitored.

2.8 MANAGEMENT OF PRE-OPERATIVE CONDITIONS

CARDIOVASCULAR DISEASE

Hypertension

- Hypertensive patients undergo a greater fall in arterial pressure on induction of anaesthesia than non-hypertensive patients.
- The patient's usual anti-hypertensive agents should be **continued** on the day of surgery (excluding ACE inhibitors and angiotensin II receptor blockers).
- Anti-hypertensive agents commonly increase the hypotensive activity of anaesthetic agents, but the intra-operative risks of a patient with untreated hypertension are much greater.
- Patients with untreated severe hypertension must be treated pre-operatively with an anti-hypertensive agent. Patients with mild to moderate hypertension may benefit from pre-treatment.

Ischaemic heart disease

- Risk should be stratified using the Goldman risk index, 12-lead ECG, echocardiography and chest radiograph.
- Patients who have well-controlled symptoms prior to surgery are rarely a problem for the anaesthetist.
- Patients with poorly controlled disease or unstable angina benefit from a short pre-operative period of treatment with a β-blocker or calcium channel antagonist.
- Patients may be treated with transdermal glyceryl trinitrate.

Arrhythmias

- Infrequent ectopic beats and nodal rhythm are common, not usually significant and require no pre-operative treatment.
- **Atrial fibrillation** (in particular fast atrial fibrillation) requires pre-operative treatment.
- **Heart block** often necessitates a pacemaker pre-operatively.

Valvular disease

- Each valve can pose different problems for the anaesthetist, so an echocardiograph is imperative in patients with suspected valve disease prior to surgery.
  - **Aortic valve**:
    - Stenosis: fixed cardiac output, ventricular arrhythmias. Peripheral vasodilation caused by general and regional anaesthesia reduces myocardial perfusion.
    - Regurgitation: cardiac failure and decreased myocardial reserve.
  - **Mitral valve**:
    - Stenosis: atrial fibrillation, pulmonary oedema and fixed cardiac output.
    - Regurgitation: pulmonary oedema, fixed cardiac output.
  - **Tricuspid valve**:
    - Usually due to disease of the other valves.
  - **Pulmonary valve**:
    - Stenosis: usually as a part of Fallot's tetralogy.
- Guidance from the National Institute for Health and Clinical Excellence no longer recommends antibiotic prophylaxis for valvular disease.

RESPIRATORY DISEASE

Asthma

- Frequency of attacks and peak expiratory flow rate (PEFR) measurements will indicate the severity of the patient's asthma.
- Patients with recent exacerbations of asthma who have changed their medications or had a reduction in their PEFR should have elective surgery postponed.
- Patients requiring emergency surgery should be given nebulized β_2 adrenoreceptor agonists (salbutamol) and steroids if necessary to optimize their respiratory function.
- If a general anaesthetic is necessary, drugs that trigger histamine release (such as propofol) may be avoided (although propofol itself is a bronchodilator and is safe for use for non-atopic asthmatics).

Chronic obstructive pulmonary disease

- Patients with severely obstructed airways are occasionally admitted to hospital early in order to receive physiotherapy and regular bronchodilators. This should improve their condition for surgery, and can be monitored by spirometry.
- General anaesthetic should be avoided if possible in these patients in favour of a regional technique.

Other respiratory problems

- Respiratory tract infections (RTIs) and recently stopping smoking can cause the bronchi to become hyper-reactive for several weeks, especially in asthmatics. Pre-operative RTIs also put the patient at risk of developing a post-operative RTI, which can be severe and potentially life-threatening.
- Patients with RTIs should have elective surgery postponed for 4 weeks.
- Draining a pneumothorax should be considered prior to surgery, although general anaesthetic techniques do exist for patients with pneumothoraces.

GASTROINTESTINAL DISEASE

Gastro-oesophageal reflux disease/hiatus hernia

- There is an increased risk of post-operative aspiration of gastric contents.
- This risk can be reduced by:
  - inducing the patient using a rapid sequence induction;
  - administering an H_2 antagonist prior to surgery.

ENDOCRINE DISEASE

Diabetes mellitus

- Tight control of diabetes mellitus (DM) prior to and during surgery is imperative and insulin must be administered to patients with type 1 diabetes even when they have been starved.
- Patients with diabetes, regardless of their treatment, must have their blood sugar monitored regularly prior to surgery as hypoglycaemia can lead to irreversible brain damage.
- For major surgery a glucose–insulin–potassium (GIK) infusion regime is followed such as a sliding scale insulin infusion.
- For any surgery, patients with insulin-dependent diabetes should receive a GIK infusion.
- Patients on oral treatment for type 2 DM should stop taking their medication 12–24 hours prior to surgery.
- The release of glucocorticoids during the 'stress response' to surgery means that patients with type 1 DM will require more insulin than normal and patients with type 2 DM may require insulin peri- and immediately post-operatively.

MICRO-facts

Sliding scale insulin infusions

Sliding scales are continuous infusions of glucose and insulin ($\pm$ potassium), the rates of which are guided by regular samples of the patient's blood glucose.

Thyroid disease

- Thyroid hormones play an important part in the regulation of metabolism; therefore, severe thyroid dysfunction increases peri-operative risk.
- Elective surgery should be postponed until patients are euthyroid.
- For urgent cases, patients should be treated with β-blockers, steroids and anti-thyroid medications to reduce risk.
- A patient with goitre should have a chest radiograph or CT to rule out tracheal deviation or mediastinal involvement.

RENAL DISEASE

Chronic renal failure

- Classified as grades 1–5 according to estimated glomerular filtration rate.
- Fluid balance must be assessed carefully prior to anaesthesia.
- Patients on haemodialysis should be selected for surgery 24 hours after their last dialysis, as their urea and electrolytes tend to be disturbed prior to this.
- LMWHs are excreted by the kidneys. Therefore, patients with renal disease need a dose adjustment to prevent bleeding.

HAEMATOLOGICAL DISORDERS

Anaemia

- Patients with severe anaemia or high expected blood loss should undergo transfusion prior to surgery.
- For patients who refuse blood transfusion, elective surgery should be postponed until they have been treated with iron and recombinant erythropoietin (cell saver devices may also be used peri-operatively).

Clotting disorders

- Clotting abnormalities should be corrected if possible prior to surgery.
- The treatment should be aimed at the cause, commonly:
  - cholestatic disorders;
  - cirrhosis leading to reduced/loss of clotting factor synthesis;
  - thrombocytopenia;
  - use of anti-coagulants, e.g. warfarin in emergency patients.
- Inherited factor deficiencies may be corrected by giving specific clotting factor concentrates.
- Patients with clotting deficiencies due to cirrhosis or other forms of liver failure would be treated with vitamin K. If this is unsuccessful (INR does not fall below 1.5 in time for surgery and platelet count not above 50×10^9/L), continuous fresh frozen plasma may be given throughout the operation.

NEUROLOGICAL DISORDERS

- Suxamethonium must be avoided in progressive neurological disorders, such as multiple sclerosis or motor neurone disease, as it can cause a dangerous rise in potassium levels.

2.9 REDUCTION OF ASPIRATION RISK

NIL BY MOUTH

- The goal of starving patients prior to surgery is to reduce the stomach contents sufficiently to reduce risk of aspiration-induced asphyxia or pneumonitis.
- For most patients:
  - no solid food for 6 hours;
  - no milky drinks for 4 hours;
  - no clear fluids for 2 hours.
- Some patients require intravenous fluids if they are to be starved:
  - Dehydration or hypoglycaemia can occur in children, patients who have taken a bowel preparation or who are pyrexial.
  - Risk of thrombosis is high in patients with sickle cell disease, polycythaemia or cyanotic heart disease.
  - Hepatorenal syndrome can be induced in patients with jaundice.

MICRO-print

Hepatorenal syndrome (HRS) is a rapid decrease in renal function in patients with cirrhosis or fulminant liver disease. Returning liver function to normal (by transplantation) will also correct renal function. Untreated HRS can be rapidly fatal.

CONSIDERATION OF RAPID SEQUENCE INDUCTION

In patients with a particularly increased risk of aspiration, a rapid sequence induction may be considered. See MICRO-facts box in Section 3.1.

MICRO-facts

Note Patients who are nil by mouth are still able to have small infrequent sips of water, especially if they need to take medications orally.

Pre-operative

2.10 INFORMED CONSENT

> ### MICRO-facts
>
> **Assessing capacity**
> Patients must be able to:
> **1.** understand the information;
> **2.** retain the information and relay it back;
> **3.** use the information to make a decision;
> **4.** communicate that decision.

Informed consent is a requirement for any medical procedure and aims to protect patient autonomy.

Gaining informed consent can be broken down into three parts: assessing capacity, giving the information and documentation.

ASSESSING CAPACITY

- Patients can lack capacity to consent for medical procedures for many reasons. Some of the most common are dementia, immaturity (legally, you are said to lack capacity to consent to a procedure if you are under 16 years old – unless Gillick competent) and some psychiatric illnesses.
- Patients with difficulty communicating decisions do not lack capacity (e.g. deafness or dysarthria).
- Capacity is commonly questioned when the patient and doctor disagree on the best course of action. Patients should be referred for an assessment of capacity based on an unprejudiced evaluation of their behaviour. Patients have the right to make a medically inadvisable decision if they are fully informed.

GIVING THE INFORMATION

- Patients must have a full understanding of the procedure, including potential alternatives, e.g. doing nothing.
- The common and serious side-effects should be explained to the patient. It is unethical to downplay the serious risks to persuade a patient to undergo a procedure.

DOCUMENTATION

- Patients must have demonstrated that they both **understand** what will happen and are able to **retain this knowledge**. This can be demonstrated by asking the patient to summarize what you have said and asking if he or she has any questions.
- Only then can the patient sign the consent form. This discussion should also be documented in the notes.

MICRO-print

Jehovah's Witnesses

- Jehovah's Witnesses are a key example of patients who may refuse therapeutic agents.
- Many (but not all) of these patients believe that accepting blood or blood products is a violation of biblical injunction and therefore refuse them on religious grounds.
- Any patient who has capacity to refuse a procedure is at liberty to do so. Ignoring a patient's decision while they are anaesthetized is unlawful and there are likely to be severe legal ramifications.
- A discussion with the patient prior to surgery should include what blood support he or she will accept. This should be clearly documented in the patient's notes. Anyone who feels unable to carry out the patient's wishes should refer him or her to an alternative practitioner.
- Blood-scavenging techniques should be used during surgery.
- Blood loss should be treated with fluids rather than with blood or plasma.
- Patients may be willing to receive iron and erythropoietin pre-operatively.
- Legal issues surrounding paediatric patients who are Jehovah's Witness are less clear cut.
- Many hospitals employ a Jehovah's Witness advocate to provide guidance on ethical matters.
- There is a specific form that records which products the patient will accept (usually available via the advocate).

MICRO-case

Mr R is a 35 year old man who is admitted for elective surgical debridement of a large right-sided groin abscess. Mr R is a large man, who drinks excessively and has been on a methadone programme for the last month after 15 years of intravenous drug abuse. The procedure is short but must be done under general anaesthesia.

The anaesthetist looking after Mr R decides that it would be safer to intubate than use a laryngeal mask airway because of Mr R's alcoholism and large size. After half an hour trying to gain intravenous access, Mr R is induced using twice the normal amount of propofol. While the anaesthetist tries to visualize Mr R's larynx by laryngoscopy, several of his teeth are damaged and one is knocked out. Intubation is successful and the operation is uneventful.

continued...

Pre-operative

continued...

While on the post-operative ward round, Mr R informs the team looking after him that he intends to sue for the dental damage, as he was not told that it was a risk prior to surgery.

Points to consider:

- Pre-operative assessment of dentition is important.
- It must be documented that patients have been warned about potential risks, such as damage to teeth.
- Patients who are likely to have loose teeth/poor dentition should be examined more carefully.
- Dental care will normally be provided to patients when healthy dentition has been damaged during airway manipulation.

Part **II**

Practice of anaesthesia

3 In the anaesthetic room

3.1 INTRODUCTION

- Techniques and medications used to produce the state of anaesthesia vary depending upon:
    - the anaesthetist's preferences and area of expertise;
    - the type and duration of surgery;
    - the health of the patient (current and previous).

The induction of a general anaesthetic should bring the patient from an alert and conscious state to one in which the patient is completely unaware of sensory

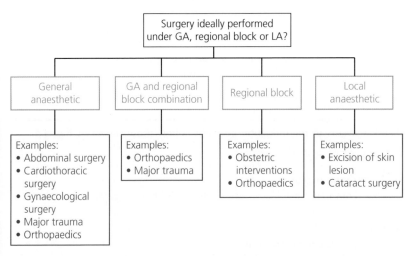

Fig. 3.1 Broad anaesthetic decision-making. GA, general anaesthetic; LA, local anaesthetic.

stimuli and is unable to create new memories. This should be achieved rapidly, calmly and painlessly, the patient's safety remaining paramount throughout the procedure.

The induction process will vary according to the type of surgery performed and the starvation status of the patient.

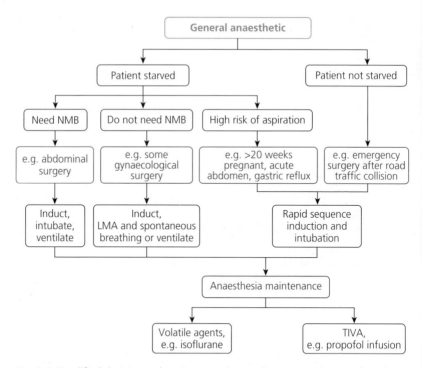

Fig. 3.2 Simplified decision-making in general anaesthesia. LMA, laryngeal mask airway; NMB, neuromuscular blocker; TIVA, total intravenous anaesthetic.

3.2 INDUCTION

The key events in the induction generally follow those shown in Fig. 3.3.

PRE-ANAESTHETIC CHECKS

- **Anaesthetic machine**:
    - comprehensive checks are made, by both an anaesthetist and a practitioner to ensure the machine is safe for use.
- **Patient**:
    - **Patient identification**.
    - **Allergy status**/could the patient be **pregnant?**
    - **Temperature**: hypothermia ($<36°C$) is a relative contraindication to anaesthesia as it poses a higher risk of bleeding and post-operative shivering.
    - **Operation specifics**: the surgery to be undertaken and, if required, what site and side is to be operated on.
    - **Confirm starvation**: the patient should not have had anything to eat or drink (clear fluids) for 6 and 2 hours respectively.

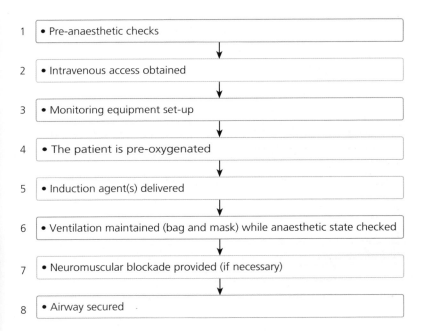

1 • Pre-anaesthetic checks

2 • Intravenous access obtained

3 • Monitoring equipment set-up

4 • The patient is pre-oxygenated

5 • Induction agent(s) delivered

6 • Ventilation maintained (bag and mask) while anaesthetic state checked

7 • Neuromuscular blockade provided (if necessary)

8 • Airway secured

Fig. 3.3 Progress of events in an induction.

MICRO-facts

Note that the **World Health Organization safety checklist** is a mandatory part of the patient's journey from pre-assessment to post-operative care. This is a document which must accompany the patient to theatre from the assessment unit/ward. More information on exactly what the checklist covers can be found at: http://www.who.int/patientsafety/safesurgery/ss_checklist/en/index.html

INTRAVENOUS ACCESS OBTAINED

- **Superficial vein cannulation**: if an intravenous (IV) induction agent is to be used, IV access must be acquired at this stage:
  - If an inhaled agent is to be used IV access may be obtained after the patient is anaesthetized. This approach is often used in paediatric cases.
  - Superficial veins on the back of the hand (dorsal metacarpal), forearm (basilic and cephalic) or at the antecubital fossa are used.
  - Cannulae come in five different sizes or 'gauges' (Table 3.1). The smaller the gauge the larger the bore (diameter) of the cannula.

> ## MICRO-facts
>
> Gauge and bore are **NOT** the same. A large bore will be a small gauge cannula and vice versa.

Table 3.1 Cannula gauge and flow rate

CANNULA GAUGE (COLOUR)	APPROX. FLOW RATE OF CRYSTALLOID FLUID (L/H)
14G (orange)	16.2
16G (grey)	10.8
18G (green)	4.8
20G (pink)	3.2
22G (blue)	1.9

MICRO-techniques
Cannulation

1. Explain procedure to the patient.
2. Identify and prepare the site (apply tourniquet proximally, apply antiseptic wipe as per hospital protocol). Lidocaine (0.2 mL of 1%) can be applied.
3. The puncture site should ideally be just distal to the union of two tributaries; if not, then just to one side of the vein.
4. Stretch skin distally and insert the needle (bevel edge facing upwards) through the skin just distal to the confluence of tributaries or just superficial and to the side of the vein.
5. Tilt the needle up to observe where the needle tip lies in relation to the vein.
6. Match the angle of the long axis of the needle with the vein and advance into the lumen.
7. If entry is successful (blood appears in the reservoir – 'first flashback'), steady the hub of the cannula then withdraw the needle while advancing the cannula. Observe for blood appearing in the plastic sheath ('second flashback') confirming that the cannula is still in the lumen.
8. Before fully removing the needle, occlude the proximal lumen of the vein/end of the cannula using mild pressure from a fingertip to reduce blood leak before the cap is connected (this is when three hands are particularly useful).
9. Place the needle in the sharps bin.
10. Check patency with 5 mL 0.9% saline/connect the infusion set.
11. Apply dressings as per hospital protocol.
12. Document the procedure as per hospital protocol.

- **Central venous cannulation**:
  - Usually obtained *after* the patient is anaesthetized.
  - For cardiovascular monitoring/delivery of certain drugs.
  - Performed using aseptic technique and ultrasound guidance to view the vessels.
  - Most commonly the internal jugular vein is used:
    - highest success rate, low complication rate;
    - right side preferable: straighter approach to superior vena cava and lower pleural apex;
    - tilt the head down to reduce the risk of air embolus and increase the size of the vein;
    - the subclavian vein can also be used.
  - Supra- or infraclavicular routes can be used but are more difficult.

MICRO-techniques

Seldinger technique for central intravenous cannulation

1. Administer local anaesthetic.
2. Locate the vein using ultrasound and insert the needle.
3. Remove the syringe to check the location (haemodynamic monitoring or observing pulsatile flow).
4. Occlude the needle to stop bleeding and prevent air embolus.
5. Advance the guidewire through the needle into the vessel.
6. Remove the needle while holding the guidewire firmly in position.
7. Enlarge the puncture site with scalpel and dilator.
8. Thread the tip of the catheter into the vessel using the guidewire to the final position, then remove the guidewire. Confirm the pressure within the vessel and compare with arterial pressure (to ensure that you are not in an artery).
9. Check the lumen position by aspirating through pigtails.
10. Suture in place and apply a dressing.
11. Check tip placement with a chest radiograph.

MONITORING EQUIPMENT SET-UP

Monitoring starts before the induction agent is given and continues until the patient has fully recovered from the anaesthetic. Monitoring serves to measure and record deviations from normal and pre-warn of adverse events. The extent of monitoring depends on a range of factors; for example, the type of operation and the current health of the patient.

Practice of anaesthesia

> ## MICRO-facts
>
> **Monitor**: a measuring instrument that is able to warn (through sounding an alarm/flashing) when the variable being measured moves outside preset values.

- **Monitoring in all patients**:
  - ECG;
  - non-invasive blood pressure;
  - pulse oximeter;
  - capnography;
  - vapour concentration analysis;
  - inspired oxygen concentration;
  - airway pressure.
- **Monitoring in some patients**:
  - peripheral nerve stimulator;
  - temperature monitor;
  - blood glucose monitoring;
  - acid–base monitoring;
  - invasive monitoring such as arterial line, central venous line, pulmonary arterial catheterization, catheter for urine output, coagulation testing, haemoglobin and electrolyte testing.

Monitoring must only ever supplement clinical observation, which should include frequently assessing:

- **Oxygenation**:
  - skin, mucous membrane and blood colour.
- **Respiration**:
  - rate, effort and reservoir bag movement.
- **Circulation**:
  - pulse: rate, rhythm and character;
  - vein filling;
  - capillary refill;
  - skin turgor;
  - temperature;
  - urine output if catheterized.
- **Depth of anaesthesia**:
  - pupils;
  - lacrimation;
  - sweating;
  - muscle movement.

PATIENT IS PRE-OXYGENATED

- After the induction agent is given respiratory effort will rapidly decrease and apnoea may occur.
- Pre-oxygenation allows for an apnoeic period in which to secure the airway – this should be short, but pre-oxygenating 'buys' time for difficulties.
- The volume in the lungs after passive expiration is the functional residual capacity (FRC). In atmospheric air, this volume (~ 2400 mL) is mostly nitrogen.
- The FRC prevents hypoxaemia during brief periods of breath-holding.
- Pre-oxygenation replaces nitrogen in the FRC with oxygen, thereby significantly increasing the length of time a patient can be apnoeic before hypoxaemia occurs.

MICRO-techniques
PRE-OXYGENATION

- Before the induction agent is given, the patient breathes 100% oxygen via a well-fitting face mask for 3 minutes, or until the oxygen concentration in expired gas exceeds 85%.
- In an emergency situation this can be replaced by the patient taking four vital capacity breaths.

INDUCTION AGENT DELIVERY

- **IV agents**:
  - General anaesthesia is most commonly induced by an IV agent.
  - Propofol is often preferred as it rapidly causes loss of consciousness and depression of pharyngeal reflexes.
- **Inhaled agents**:
  - Usually sevoflurane is used as it is the least unpleasant and irritant to inhale.
  - Delivered by gradually increasing the concentration in oxygen with or without the addition of nitrous oxide.
- **Intramuscular**:
  - Ketamine can be given intramuscularly (mainly used in pre-hospital anaesthesia).
- **Adjunctive agents**:
  - In conjunction with one of the above, an opiate (e.g. fentanyl/ remifentanil) and/or a benzodiazepine (e.g. midazolam) shortens induction times, provides intra-operative analgesia, reduces cardiovascular depression by the induction agent and (in the case of benzodiazepines) produces amnesia. See the 'Six As' on p. 45.

VENTILATION MAINTAINED

- After delivery of the induction agent the patient will rapidly lose consciousness and airway patency. Except in the case of rapid sequence induction prior to securing the airway with the appropriate adjunct, the patient can be ventilated using the bag–valve–mask technique.

NEUROMUSCULAR BLOCKADE

- Some patients are paralysed, using a neuromuscular blocker.

AIRWAY SECURED

- Using airway adjuncts such as an endotracheal tube or a laryngeal mask airway.

MICRO-facts

- Rapid sequence intubation can be used in patients who are at increased risk of aspiration, e.g. emergency cases who have not been fasted.
- It is aimed at reducing the time from unconsciousness (and subsequent loss of airway security) to intubation (and securing of the airway).
- The key differences are that a short-acting NMB is administered in rapid succession to the induction agent. The patient is then intubated without the use of manual ventilation, prior to inflation of the cuff. Manual pressure is applied to the cricoid cartilage (the 'Sellick manoeuvre') prior to intubation to further reduce aspiration risk.

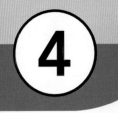

4 Airways and ventilation

4.1 AIRWAYS

One of the cornerstones of anaesthesia is airway management. During general anaesthesia or in emergency life-support situations, patients often require help in maintaining an open route for oxygen to reach the lungs, while preventing aspiration of stomach contents. The importance of airway patency cannot be overstressed: it is always the first thing that should be assessed in any acutely ill patient.

> **MICRO-reference**
> For up-to-date basic life support guidelines: www.resus.org.uk

ASSESSMENT OF THE AIRWAY

- **Look**:
    - for a foreign body (and remove if possible);
    - for chest wall movements.
- **Listen**:
    - for breath sounds;
    - for sounds of obstruction (wheeze/stridor).
- **Feel**:
    - for air flow at the mouth;
    - for chest movements.
      This should take no longer than 10 seconds.

BASIC AIRWAY MANOEUVRES

- Intended to move the tongue forward to prevent occlusion of the pharynx/larynx.
    - **Head tilt chin lift**: flexion of the lower cervical spine and extension of the head at the atlantoaxial joint tilts the head backwards moving the tongue away from the pharynx. This can be known as 'sniffing the morning air' (this manoeuvre is performed only when the cervical spine is known to be intact).

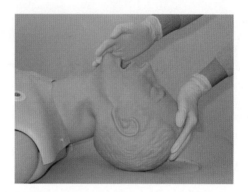

Fig. 4.1 Chin lift.

- **Jaw thrust**: the most effective airway manoeuvre, which can also be used in patients with cervical injury with the help of in-line head stabilization. The posterior aspect of the mandible is thrust forwards.

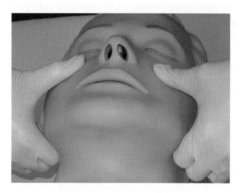

Fig. 4.2 Jaw thrust.

- **Clearance of secretions/regurgitations**: the airways can become blocked by secretions/vomit:
    - **Suction**: secretions can be removed from the upper airways using suction.
    - **Recovery position**: when suction is not available, the patient can be placed in the recovery position, which facilitates drainage of fluids from the mouth and therefore reduces the risk of aspiration.

AIRWAY ADJUNCTS

Various artificial devices are available which can be used to keep the airway open:

- **Guedel airway** (or oropharyngeal airway):
    - A simple C-shaped tube that comes in various sizes that is used to prevent the tongue from covering the epiglottis.

- The size is chosen by measuring in profile from the mouth to the angle of the jaw.
- The airway can then be inserted while inverted, then rotated 180° while advancing over the tongue.
- This can stimulate the gag reflex in conscious patients – if it does, take it out!
- **Nasopharyngeal airway**:
  - A tube with a flared end (to keep the external end of the tube outside the patient's nose) passed down through the nose into the pharynx to bypass the tongue.
  - This cannot be used in base of skull fractures because of the risk of insertion into the cranial cavity – check for Battle's sign (mastoid ecchymosis), racoon eyes, cerebrospinal fluid otorrhoea/rhinorrhoea, cranial nerve palsy etc.

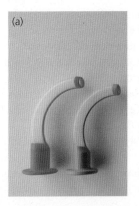
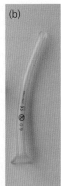

(a)

(b)

Fig. 4.3 (a) Guedel and (b) nasopharyngeal airways.

MICRO-facts

After introduction of any airway, patency should be checked by visualizing chest wall movement and by auscultating both lungs.

- **Laryngeal mask airway** (LMA):
  - This is a tube inserted through the pharynx with a small mask designed to cover the larynx. The mask is then inflated to cause a seal (if in place the tube should move upwards slightly on inflation). i-gel LMAs are also available that do not require inflation.
  - An LMA can be used for both spontaneous and controlled ventilation, and can also be used for surgery when the risk of aspiration is very low

(e.g. in gynaecological or orthopaedic day case surgery on fully starved and otherwise healthy individuals).
- When removing, it is important not to deflate the cuff of the LMA, so secretions from the upper airways are removed on the rim of the mask.

DEFINITIVE AIRWAYS

Endotracheal (ET) tube

- The definitive airway. It provides a secure, patent airway while the inflated cuff forms an airtight seal preventing aspiration of stomach contents.
- In an 'easy' intubation, the tube is inserted while visualizing the vocal cords on laryngoscopy (see Micro-techniques: Laryngoscopy):
  - For patients with a grade 1 view at laryngoscopy, the ET tube can be advanced, aiming between the vocal cords, and, with the tube in place, the cuff is inflated.
  - For patients who are more difficult (i.e. grade 2+) external laryngeal pressure can improve the view, and for those still inadequate for intubation other techniques may be employed:
    - **Bougie**: a plastic introducer, 60 cm long, 5 mm in diameter, which is used as a guide for the ET tube. Correct placement is confirmed by the 'clicks' as it passes over successive rings of cartilage in the trachea and stops once reaching the carina. The ET tube is then slid over the bougie into the trachea.
    - **Stylet**: a pre-curved stylet in the ET tube can aid placement by stiffening the tube.
    - **Lightwand**: transillumination of the neck occurs when the light is in the trachea, below thyroid cartilage but not the oesophagus.

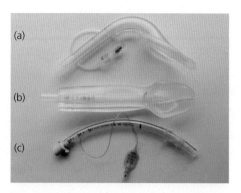

Fig. 4.4 (a) Laryngeal mask airway (b) i-gel; (c) endotracheal tube.

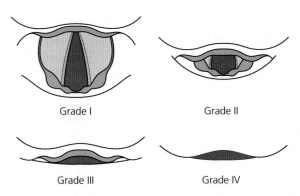

Fig. 4.5 Cormack and Lehane grading of the view of the vocal cords at laryngoscopy.

MICRO-techniques
LARYNGOSCOPY
1. The patient is placed in the 'sniffing the morning air' position – neck flexed on chest to about 35° and the head extended on the neck so that the face is tilted back 15° from horizontal.
2. When using a Macintosh laryngoscope, the blade is inserted to the right side of the mouth so the flange of the blade moves the tongue over to the left
as the blade is advanced centrally towards the base of the tongue.
3. Lifting the blade exposes the epiglottis.
4. Advancing further with continued lifting exposes the vocal cords (grade 1).
5. In more difficult patients laryngoscopy will reveal less and can be graded as such (Table 4.1).

Table 4.1 Laryngoscopic grading

GRADING OF THE VIEW AT LARYNGOSCOPY BY CORMACK AND LEHANE	
Grade 1	Vocal cords visualized
Grade 2	Posterior portion of the laryngeal opening visualized
Grade 3	Epiglottis visualized
Grade 4	Only soft palate visualized

From Cormack R., Lehane J. Difficult tracheal intubation in obstetrics. *Anaesthesia*. 1984; **39**: 1105–11.

Practice of anaesthesia

- **Alternative laryngoscope blades**: various blades are available in addition to the standard Macintosh laryngoscope.
- **Video-assisted airway management**: video feed allows visualization of the vocal cords in more difficult-to-intubate patients.

- **Nasotracheal (NT) tube**:
  - More secure than an ET tube but more technically challenging and higher complication rate. Used mainly for oral surgery.

Emergency airways (cricothyroidotomy)

- Occasionally used in life-threatening emergencies to bypass obstruction. Needle cricothyroidotomy involves inserting a dilator and then a reasonably large-bore airway into the trachea. Techniques involving non-specialized kit, for example cannulae, can be employed in an emergency but are discouraged.

Surgical airways (tracheotomy)

- Involves creating a direct airway by incisions on the anterior aspect of the neck and trachea. The stoma created can be used as an airway with or without the use of a tracheostomy tube.
- Can be elective (e.g. for long-term intensive therapy patients or extensive head and neck surgery) or emergency (e.g. for massive facial trauma or head and neck tumours).

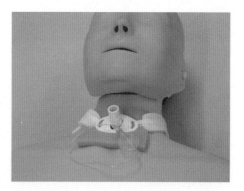

Fig. 4.6 Tracheostomy *in situ*.

MICRO-case

A 69 year old man with a body mass index of 35 and a mass in his neck is found unconscious and cyanotic by a nurse shortly after his dinner. He is breathing spontaneously but with slow gasps and marked stridor; his O_2 saturation is 75% and he has a heart rate of 70 beats/min. Using an ABC approach, the house officer performs airway manoeuvres, inserts a

continued...

continued...

Guedel airway and commences bag–valve–mask ventilation with 100% oxygen and manages to improve the saturations to 85%. However, the stridor persists despite suction removing some of the patient's soup from his throat. The patient's saturations continue to fall and his heart rate rises to 85 beats/min.

The crash team that had been called arrives shortly after and the anaesthetist performs urgent tracheal intubation, securing the airway using a 6 mm cuffed endotracheal (ET) tube. She comments that, although the patient's vocal cords were easy to visualize, she encountered significant resistance when passing the ET tube beyond them. The saturations quickly increase to 98% and shortly after the patient becomes haemodynamically stable.

The patient is transferred to the intensive therapy unit and is conscious and responsive with mechanical ventilation. After a CT scan shows that the tumour is responsible for the airway obstruction, a plan is made to treat the suspected lymphoma with chemotherapy.

Points to consider:

- In any acutely ill patient, use the ABC approach.
- Call for help in a peri-arrest situation.
- ET intubation is the best way to secure a patient's airway – if skilled to do so. If not, a laryngeal mask airway or simple airway manoeuvres with bag and mask ventilation are safer, as the main goal is maintaining oxygenation.

4.2 VENTILATION

In addition to a patent airway, adequate ventilation is necessary to allow adequate perfusion of tissues. If spontaneous ventilation is either not present or inadequate, various modes of mechanical ventilation are available. These usually involve applying a positive pressure to the patient's airway to inflate the lungs.

REASONS FOR RESPIRATORY SUPPORT

- Respiratory failure:
    - the primary indication;
    - the reason patients are ventilated when under general anaesthetic;
    - usually a clinical diagnosis; indicators include respiratory rate (high or low), exhaustion, laboured breathing, hypoxia and hypercarbia.
- Airway protection.
- Control of intra-cranial pressure.

POSITIVE PRESSURE VENTILATION

- Ideal characteristics of a mechanical ventilator:
    - provide appropriate ventilation modes;

Practice of anaesthesia

- simple and practical to use;
- reliable;
- monitoring and alarms;
- easy to keep aseptic.

Ventilator phases and cycling

- **Inspiration phase**:
  - During the inspiration phase either a flow rate or pressure can be generated by a ventilator to fill the patient's lungs.
  - Pressures created by flow generators will vary according to the patient's respiratory mechanics (see Chapter 1, Physiology).
  - Flow rates created by pressure generators also vary according to the patient's respiratory mechanics:
    - Inspiratory cycling: i.e. when to end the inspiratory phase and commence the expiratory phase; can be set to a volume, pressure or time.
- **Expiration phase**:
  - Expiration is often passive, reducing the pressure or flow to nothing to allow the lungs to deflate.
  - Alternatively, positive end-expiratory pressure (PEEP) can be used; this allows the lungs to deflate but prevents the relative pressure from reaching zero, thereby increasing the functional residual capacity.
    - Expiratory cycling:
      - In other words, when to end the expiratory phase and commence the inspiratory phase.
      - Usually timed, often controlling the inspiration to expiration ratio.
      - Alternatively, some ventilators are able to detect when a patient is initiating a breath (e.g. synchronized intermittent mandatory ventilation (SIMV)) and support it.

Modes of respiratory support

- **Bag–valve–mask**:
  - The simplest method of ventilation – used frequently in resuscitation situations (and prior to the use of mechanical ventilation in anaesthetized patients).
  - When the bag is squeezed, air or oxygen is forced through the one-way valve and the flexible mask into the patient's lungs.
  - The mask needs a tight seal with the patient's face while airway manoeuvres are performed. This is easier with two people but can be performed with one hand holding the bag and the other holding the

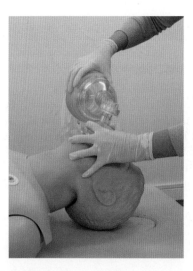

Fig. 4.7 Bag and mask ventilation.

mask to the patient's face with the thumb, index and middle finger while performing a jaw thrust with the little finger.

- **Intermittent positive pressure ventilation** (IPPV):
  - positive pressure delivered intermittently via ET or NT tube to inflate the lungs.
- **Non-invasive positive pressure ventilation** (NIPPV):
  - positive pressure delivered intermittently via a tight-fitting face/nasal mask to inflate the lungs.
- **Controlled mechanical ventilation**:
  - ventilation determined solely by machine settings;
  - used on apnoeic patients (e.g. in theatre with neuromuscular blockade).
- **Assisted mechanical ventilation**:
  - The ventilator supports the patient's spontaneous inspiration and assists by supplying intermittent positive pressure.
  - There are several types:
    - **Intermittent mandatory ventilation**: the ventilator performs IPPV breaths but allows the patient to breathe spontaneously in between.
    - **SIMV**: the ventilator recognizes the patient's breaths and provides supplementary synchronized IPPV, but will provide extra mandatory breaths if there are periods of apnoea.
    - **Assisted spontaneous breaths (ASV)/pressure support ventilation**: the ventilator supplements each spontaneous breath with a preset pressure level – can be combined with SIMV.

Practice of anaesthesia

- **PEEP**:
    - A baseline positive pressure level is supplied with IPPV during expiration.
    - This increases the FRC, and increases the compliance at the start of inspiration.
    - It can prevent distal airway collapse and keeps alveoli inflated during expiration, thereby improving oxygenation.
    - It increases intra-thoracic pressure, decreasing venous return and ultimately blood pressure.
- **Continuous positive airways pressure**:
    - Essentially non-invasive PEEP, used in spontaneously breathing patients.
    - Used to improve SaO_2 and also as a treatment for pulmonary oedema.

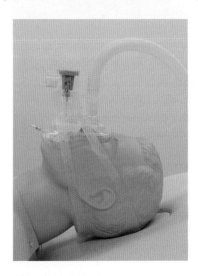

Fig. 4.8 Continuous positive airways pressure.

- **Bilevel positive airways pressure (BiPAP)**:
    - BiPAP = NIPPV + ASV.
    - Provides PEEP plus an increased pressure during inspiration.
    - Used to support patients with obstruction and those with respiratory failure before more invasive respiratory support.
- **Negative-pressure ventilator**:
    - More closely resembles spontaneous breathing.
    - **Iron lung**:
        - The patient is placed in a sealed chamber providing intermittent negative ventilation.

- However, because of the inconvenience of its size and the patient's inaccessibility, it is now obsolete compared with positive pressure systems and is very rarely used.

Note These modes of ventilation are not mutually exclusive and many can be used in conjunction with others.

5 Oxygen

Oxygen is one of the most important drugs used in hospital. While widely available and lifesaving when used appropriately, it is often administered without properly considering the risks and benefits. Monitoring of patients receiving oxygen therapy is also very important.

- Limited stores of oxygen in the body mean that:
    - tissue hypoxia will occur within roughly 4 minutes after failure of ventilation, gas exchange or circulation;
    - effective oxygen administration (increasing the fraction of inspired oxygen (FiO_2)) increases oxygen transport by increasing the saturation of haemoglobin.

5.1 INITIATING OXYGEN THERAPY

> **MICRO-facts**
>
> In the acute setting, inadequate delivery of oxygen carries a far higher risk of death and disability than the relatively low risks associated with high-dose oxygen.

ACUTE SETTING

- In acute conditions the aim of oxygen therapy is to provide high levels of oxygen to preserve life while the underlying pathology is resolved.
- Initiation of oxygen therapy is one of the first things to be considered for an acutely ill patient, often started as part of the ABC assessment.
- High-dose oxygen should be given with care in patients who have chronic obstructive pulmonary disease (COPD) with type II respiratory failure (high CO_2; affects 10–15% of patients with COPD) as high O_2 can, in CO_2 retention, lead to respiratory acidosis. However, it is important to bear in mind that **hypoxaemia will kill the patient before CO_2 retention will. Therefore, give high-flow O_2 and then do a blood gas.**

5.2 ADMINISTERING OXYGEN

Delivery can be divided into **low-flow** and **high-flow** systems. While high-flow masks deliver enough flow to provide for peak inspiratory flow, low-flow masks deliver a proportion. Non-rebreather systems can allow very high levels of inspired oxygen.

LOW-FLOW SYSTEMS

- Include basic face masks and nasal cannulae (note that FiO_2 is lower for equivalent flow rates via nasal cannulae).

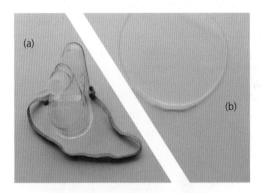

Fig. 5.1 (a) Simple facemask and (b) nasal cannula.

- These supply a flow of oxygen which supplements normal air. Thus, the FiO_2 will vary depending on the ventilatory minute volume; as the minute volume increases, the oxygen supplied becomes 'diluted' in normal air and the FiO_2 decreases. For examples, see Table 5.1
- FiO_2 can be (crudely) approximated as:

$$[(\text{Oxygen flow rate}) + (\text{Air inspired} \times 0.21)]$$
$$\div (\text{Ventilatory minute volume})$$

Table 5.1 Ventilatory volume

VENTILATORY MINUTE VOLUME	OXYGEN FLOW RATE (L/MIN)	AIR INSPIRED (L)	FiO_2 (%)
Normal (5–8 litres)	0	5–8	21
Normal (5–8 litres)	2	3–6	41–53
Respiratory distress (30 litres)	2	28	26

Practice of anaesthesia

- 2 litres of oxygen with a normal ventilatory minute volume (5 L/min; i.e. 10 breaths/min at 500 mL/breath) will increase FiO_2. However, this increase will be attenuated by respiratory distress, which can be higher than 30 litres (i.e. 40 breaths/min at 750 mL/breath), can be reduced to 29%, which would not provide much benefit for the patient.
- At low flow rates, rebreathing occurs as the mask is not flushed, increasing the potential for CO_2 retention.
  - **Non-rebreather masks**:
    - include Hudson masks;
    - incorporate non-rebreathing valves and reservoir bags to collect oxygen during expiration;
    - mean the FiO_2 can be very high even when there is a high ($>60\%$) ventilatory minute volume;
    - are useful in the very acute/emergency situation, when a patient requires high levels of oxygen.

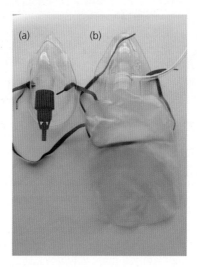

Fig. 5.2 (a) Venturi and (b) non-rebreathe face masks.

HIGH-FLOW SYSTEMS

- Include **Venturi face masks**:
  - These provide the patient with an FiO_2 independent of ventilatory minute volume as the high flow rates prevent breathing of normal air or rebreathing expired gases.
  - Venturi masks provide an accurate fixed FiO_2, up to 60%, but can alternatively be relatively low.

- The ability to provide low FiO_2 without significant rebreathing of expired gases is of use for patients who have COPD with type II respiratory failure.

MICRO-case

Mrs C is a 68 year old former office worker with known chronic obstructive pulmonary disease (COPD) who continues to smoke. She presents to the Accident and Emergency Department with increasing shortness of breath and increasing production of sputum. This has been getting worse over the past 2 days. She has no other symptoms.

On examination she sits on the edge of the bed, splinting herself and breathing with pursed lips. Her chest is wheezy and has diffuse, coarse crackles. The doctor diagnoses an infective COPD exacerbation and she is commenced on 1 litre of oxygen via nasal cannula, ipratropium and salbutamol nebulisers, co-amoxiclav and 30 mg of prednisilone.

While on the medical assessment unit, she becomes increasingly short of breath and the nurse checks her saturations, which are 83%. As a result, the doctor increases her oxygen to 2 litres and returns to do an arterial blood gas (ABG) 1 hour later. This shows a pH of 7.38, PO_2 of 6.5 and a PCO_2 of 5.45. The doctor increases her oxygen to 35%. Repeat ABG shows a pH of 7.18, PO_2 of 8.45 and a PCO_2 of 7.24 and she is still short of breath. She is commenced on a theophylline infusion. However, she fails to improve and is transferred to the intensive therapy unit for non-invasive ventilation (NIV).

After 2 days of NIV she is no longer acidotic and makes a full recovery.

Points to consider:

- O_2 is a life-saving medication; a high CO_2 will not kill your patient – hypoxia will.
- Venturi valve masks are useful in patients with COPD, as they enable a fixed amount of O_2 to be given.
- A small number of people with COPD can begin to retain CO_2 on higher levels of oxygen. The priority is to increase oxygenation, which may require different forms of respiratory support to avoid making the patient acidotic. It is important to check on patients frequently when their O_2 has been increased.

5.3 MONITORING SATURATION OF HAEMOGLOBIN WITH OXYGEN

NON-INVASIVE PULSE OXIMETRY

- Probe placed on finger/toe/ear lobe.
- Calculates saturation by measuring the pulsatile change in absorption of red and infrared light caused by the difference in colour of oxygen-bound and -unbound haemoglobin.

Practice of anaesthesia

- Measures saturation (*S*) in peripheral blood (p) of oxygen – hence SpO_2.
- Normal saturations are above 95%; saturations less than 90% suggest respiratory failure.
- Normal values for individual patients vary and patients used to low oxygenation (e.g. those with COPD) can often tolerate lower SpO_2. Often, **changes** in SpO_2 value are more useful than absolute values.
- The number of red cells in the blood cannot be determined by pulse oximetry:
    - Patients with a normal oxygen saturation, but very high numbers of red cells (such as in polycythaemia), will appear to have low O_2 saturations.
    - Conversely, severely anaemic patients in whom all the available red blood cells are saturated will appear to have normal saturations despite being hypoxic.

BLOOD GASES FROM ARTERIAL BLOOD SAMPLING (Table 5.2)

Table 5.2 Normal ranges for arterial blood with room air (21% O_2)

pH	7.35–7.45
PaO_2	11–13 kPa
$PaCO_2$	4.7–6.0 kPa
HCO_3^-	24–30 mmol/L
Base excess	−2 to +2 mmol/L
Anion gap	12–16 mmol/L

- Like many tests, having a system to interpret the values is important. One such system is described here.

Assess oxygenation

See Fig. 5.3.

Assess acid–base disturbance

See Fig. 5.4.

Consider cause of acid–base disturbance

- **Respiratory acidosis:**
    - may be the result of any cause of respiratory failure.
- **Metabolic acidosis:**
    - this can be due to reduced HCO_3^- levels directly or the presence of other acids (other than carbonic acid). By calculating the anion gap this can be elucidated.

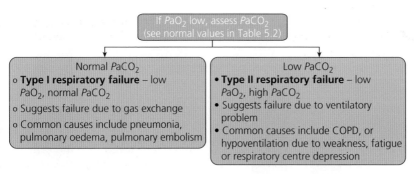

Fig. 5.3 Type I and type II respiratory failure. COPD, chronic obstructive pulmonary disease.

- **Respiratory alkalosis**:
    - this can be due to hyperventilation (anxiety/sepsis/stroke).
- **Metabolic alkalosis**:
    - common causes include losses from the gut (vomiting), hypercalcaemia, hyperaldosteronism and diuretic usage.

Anion gap (Table 5.3)

Table 5.3 Anion gap

NORMAL/LOW ANION GAP	HIGH ANION GAP
Renal tubular acidosis	Ketoacidosis
Loss of HCO_3^-, e.g. in diarrhoea	Lactic acidosis
Excess normal (0.9%) saline	Ingestion of salicylate, methanol, ethylene glycol
Drugs, e.g. acetazolamide	Renal failure

- Calculated as follows:

$$(Na^+ + K^+) - (Cl^- + HCO_3^-)$$

- Diseases affecting concentrations of these and other simple ions, e.g. calcium, magnesium and phosphate, lead to an acidosis with a low or normal anion gap.
- A high anion gap is due to the presence of acids which are not routinely measured, e.g. lactate.

Practice of anaesthesia

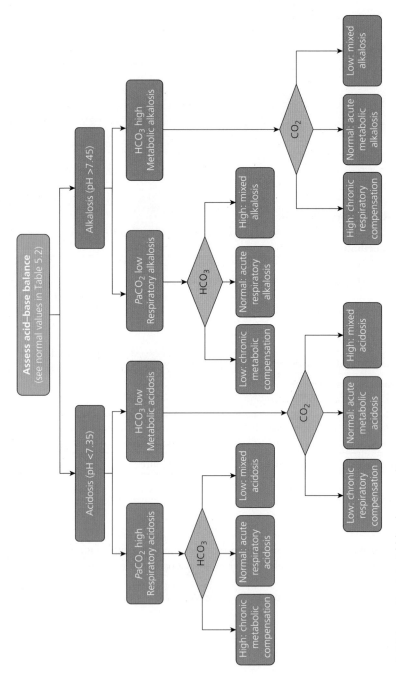

Fig. 5.4 Interpreting arterial blood gas results.

MICRO-techniques
Arterial blood gas sampling: radial artery puncture

1. Obtain informed consent, perform Allen's test and ensure the patient has no bleeding defects or infections (e.g. cellulitis) over the artery.
2. Wash your hands and wear gloves.
3. Allen's test:
   Tests patency of ulnar and radial arteries (so hand circulation is maintained if the radial artery is damaged during the procedure).
   (a) Ask the patient to make a tight clenched fist and compress the tissues over the ulnar and radial arteries.
   (b) Ask the patient to relax their hand; if you have occluded the arteries it should remain pale and unperfused.
   (c) Release one artery and observe the reperfusion of the hand demonstrating the artery's patency. Repeat, this time releasing the other artery.
   (d) Failure for one of the arteries is a *positive* Allen's test, which is a contraindication for arterial blood gas (ABG) sampling as only one artery supplies the hand.
4. **Note** that various ABG needle and syringe systems exist. Ensure that you have had training in the use of ABG sampling with the equipment you are using.
5. Palpate the radial artery along the area where it meets the wrist to find the area of maximum pulsation.
6. Clean the area of skin to be punctured. After cleaning, **do not repalpate** where you are puncturing. However, palpating slightly above/below the area can be helpful.
7. If you plan to use local anaesthetic, use 1% lidocaine.
8. Some ABG systems require that you discard heparin from the needle prior to puncturing the vessel; some will not. Additionally, some work with the plunger retracted to a given volume and some fill themselves. Check local equipment before use to prevent mistakes.
9. With the wrist flexed, insert the needle 45–90° to the skin and guide the needle to where you felt the artery.
10. The arterial pressure will fill the syringe when you have punctured the artery.
11. When filled, remove the needle and apply **firm** pressure to the site for a minimum of 5 minutes (the patient or an assistant may do this).

Practice of anaesthesia

Local and regional anaesthesia

6.1 ADVANTAGES TO REGIONAL ANAESTHESIA

Regional anaesthesia allows the patient to remain conscious; therefore, airway and ventilation management is unnecessary. It also has fewer systemic side-effects; therefore, safer for use in the patient with a large range of co-morbidities.

> **MICRO-facts**
>
> **Contraindictations to local or regional anaesthesia**
> - Patient choice.
> - Anti-coagulation or coagulopathy.
> - Untreated hypovolaemia (especially when considering spinal anaesthesia).
> - Major infection.
> - Trauma/burns over the proposed injection site.
> - Raised intra-cranial pressure.

6.2 ANAESTHESIA AND ANALGESIA WITHIN THE SPINAL COLUMN: CENTRAL NEURAL BLOCKADE

SPINAL ANAESTHESIA

- Injection of anaesthetic agent into the **intrathecal space**, directly into the cerebrospinal fluid around the lumbar region below the level of L1/2 where the spinal cord ends.
- **Indications**:
  - Surgical procedures below the level of the umbilicus.
  - **Note** that this is not used for procedures above the umbilicus because of difficulties in maintaining spontaneous ventilation while preventing painful stimuli from traction on the peritoneum and pressure on the diaphragm.

MICRO-techniques
Spinal anaesthesia
1. Establish venous access with a wide-bore cannula.
2. The patient should be in the sitting position with their feet placed down the side of the bed and their elbows resting on their thighs.
3. Find Tuffier's line: a line joining both iliac crests crossing L4.
4. Locate the L3/L4 interspace from this line.
5. Sterilize the skin.
6. Inject local anaesthesia (lidocaine) into the subcutaneous tissue.
7. Insert an introducer into the midline at 90° to the skin.
8. The needle will pass through the following:
   (a) supraspinous ligament;
   (b) interspinous ligament;
   (c) ligamentum flavum;
   (d) dura mater.
9. Cerebrospinal fluid should flow from the introducer needle.
10. Inject local anaesthetic.
11. Test for sensory block using blunt pinprick in all dermatomes. Motor loss can be estimated using the Bromage scale (Table 6.1).

Table 6.1 **Degree of motor block from spinal anaesthesia**

DEGREE OF MOTOR BLOCK	BROMAGE CRITERIA	PERCENTAGE SCORE (%)
1 No block	Full flexion of knees and feet	0
2 Partial block	Just able to flex knees Full foot movement	33
3 Almost complete	Unable to flex knees Partial foot flexion	66
4 Complete	Unable to move legs or feet	100

- **Drug doses**:
  - 3–3.25 mL of **bupivicaine** 0.5% provides block level to T6/7 for a lower abdominal operation site. Lower doses are used in obstetrics.
- **Complications**:
  - Post-dural puncture headache:
    - loss of cerebrospinal fluid through the dural puncture site leads to a low-pressure headache due to traction on the cranial meninges;
    - characteristically relieved by lying flat and exacerbated by sitting/ standing/straining;

Practice of anaesthesia

- – if severe can cause cranial nerve symptoms, i.e. alters vision and hearing;
- – ensure adequate hydration in these patients, caffeine may also be beneficial.
- Nausea and vomiting (if awake).
- Rarely, can cause nerve damage.
- **Physiological consequences** of central neural blockade that must be managed include:
  - hypotension;
  - urinary retention;
  - bradycardia.

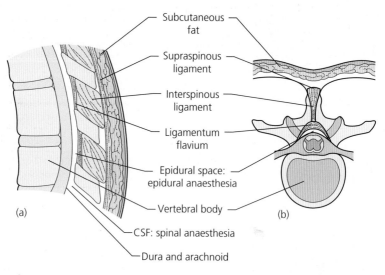

Fig. 6.1 (a and b) Anatomy for central neural blockades. CSF, cerebrospinal fluid.

EPIDURAL ANAESTHESIA

- Injection of anaesthetic agent into the epidural space.
- **Indications**:
  - usually used with additional light general anaesthetic for abominal and lower limb surgery;
  - for acute and chronic pain relief, i.e. labour pains, post-laparotomy.
- **Anatomy**: see Fig. 6.1.
  The differences between spinal and epidural anaesthesia are shown in Table 6.2.

Table 6.2 **Differences between spinal and epidural anaesthesia**

	Spinal	Epidural
Onset	2–5 minutes Rapid onset	20–30 minutes Slow onset
Duration	2–3 hours Short duration	3–5 hours Longer duration Catheter can be inserted to provide 'top-up' to extend duration by days/weeks
Drug volume	2.5–4 mL	20–30 mL
Quality	Rapid surgical anaesthesia	May be inadequate in some dermatomes
Use of spinal catheters	Spinal catheters uncommon	Catheter often inserted to allow top-up doses (via patient-controlled analgesia) or prolonged infusions
Summary	Dense anaesthetic cover provided below the umbilicus with small doses of drug	Requires larger doses of drug for less dense surgical anaesthesia. Can be used more flexibly in the lumbar and thoracic regions Duration can be extended to days/weeks by insertion of a catheter

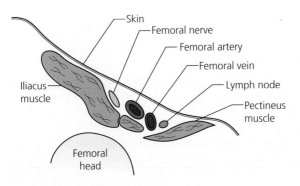

Fig. 6.2 **The femoral nerve and its surrounding anatomy.**

Practice of anaesthesia

PERIPHERAL NERVE BLOCK

- Blocking of the femoral nerve, often in combination with the sciatic, obturator and lateral cutaneous nerves.
- **Indication**: to provide pain relief for major orthopaedic surgery of the lower limb, especially to femur and knee joint, e.g. total knee replacement, cruciate ligament reconstruction.
- **Anatomy**: see Fig. 6.2.
- Procedure: see Micro-techniques: Femoral block.
- **Drug doses**:
  - 15 mL of bupivacaine 0.5% provides 12–18 hours of anaesthesia.
- **Complications**:
  - accidental injection of local anaesthetic into the femoral vessels;
  - pressure sores and immobility owing to prolonged anaesthetic;
  - intraneural injection can lead to neuritis, then on to chronic pain and disability.

MICRO-techniques
Femoral block
1. The patient lies supine.
2. Identify the inguinal ligament: the femoral pulse is immediately distal to this.
3. Locate the nerve under ultrasound guidance, approximately 1 cm lateral to pulsation of the femoral artery and 1–2 cm distal to the inguinal ligament.
4. Insert a regional block needle at 45°; pressure is felt as the needle pierces the fascia lata with a secondary 'pop' as it enters the nerve sheath.
5. Aspirate and slowly inject.
6. Use a peripheral nerve stimulator to test.

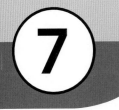

7 Drugs in the anaesthetic room

There are many different drugs in an anaesthetic room that will be used regularly, rarely, alone or in conjunction with others. Knowledge of individual agents, their pharmacology and reasons for administration is essential to understanding the art of anaesthesia. Classes of drugs discussed in this chapter are:

- general anaesthetics;
- muscle relaxants: neuromuscular blockers;
- anti-cholinesterases;
- local anaesthetics.

7.1 GENERAL ANAESTHETICS

Anaesthetic drugs can be used for induction of anaesthesia, maintenance of anaesthesia or as sedatives depending on dose. They are either given intravenously as a liquid or inhaled as a gas. For most cases intravenous (IV) agents are used for induction and inhaled agents are used for maintenance.

INTRAVENOUS ANAESTHETICS

Phenols: propofol (2,6-di-isopropylphenol)

- **Mode of action**: fast-acting lipid-soluble molecule that can rapidly cross the blood–brain barrier and, once in the cerebral circulation, causes cortical depression and loss of consciousness. Fast redistribution first to muscle and then to fat leads to rapid recovery of consciousness.
- **Speed of induction**: 30–45 seconds (one arm to brain circulation time).
- **Duration of action**: 4–7 minutes.
- **Advantages**: depresses upper airway reflexes, anti-emetic.
- **Side-effects**:
  - hypotension;
  - apnoea of up to 60 seconds;
  - respiratory depression;
  - pain on injection;
  - involuntary movements;

- hiccoughs;
- propofol infusion syndrome.
- **Elimination**: fast elimination by the liver.
- **Clinical effects**: loss of consciousness.

MICRO-facts

Propofol infusion syndrome

A triad of:

1. metabolic acidosis;
2. acute cardiomyopathy;
3. skeletal myopathy.
   This is possibly due to a failure of free fatty acid metabolism.
   Almost unknown after a single application.

- **Points to note**:
  - As speed of induction is directly related to arm–brain circulation time, it can be delayed in heart failure and shock.
  - This is a distinctive thick white solution ('milk of amnesia') containing 2% propofol in soybean oil, glycerol and purified egg phosphatide.
  - Does not accumulate. Therefore, it can be used for maintenance when repeated injections/infusions are needed; usually achieved by giving through a syringe driver.

Barbiturates: sodium thiopentone

- **Mode of action**: a weak, protein-bound acid that, when metabolized to its active form, pentobarbital, causes cortical depression.
- **Speed of induction**: 30–45 seconds (one arm to brain circulation time).
- **Advantages**: rapid, smooth induction to anaesthesia. Causes a reduction in cerebral metabolic rate of oxygen consumption, making it useful in cardiopulmonary bypass operations (although propofol is similar).
- **Side-effects**:
  - Hypotension, respiratory depression and reduced sensitivity to raised CO_2, leading to periods of transient apnoea.
  - Coughing, laryngospasm and bronchoconstriction due to poor suppression of laryngeal reflexes.
  - Pain on injection and tissue damage.
- **Elimination**: slowly by the liver.
- **Clinical effects**: loss of consciousness.
- **Points to note**:
  - has a pale yellow colour and gives the patient the taste of garlic/onions;
  - not commonly used for maintenance via IV infusion owing to its slow elimination by the liver.

Phencyclidine derivatives: ketamine

- **Mode of action**: acts on the N-methyl-d-aspartate receptor and opioid receptors to give a strong anaesthetic and analgesic effect.
- **Speed of induction**: 50–70 seconds.
- **Advantages**: causes sleep, dissociation and analgesia; does not cause respiratory depression.
- **Side-effects**:
  - Emergence phenomena: hallucinations with vivid dreams and psychosis, diplopia, temporary blindness, hypertension and tachycardia.
- **Clinical effects**: loss of consciousness and analgesia.
- **Points to note**:
  - ketamine has two stereoisomers, of which S is the more potent and has fewer unwanted side-effects;
  - not often used as IV maintenance as it has an unpleasant recovery.

Benzodiazepines: midazolam

- **Mode of action**: γ-aminobutyric acid enhancer.
- **Speed of induction**: 40–70 seconds.
- **Advantages**: lipid soluble with good blood–brain transfer. Causes sedation, hypnosis and is an anti-convulsant. It also causes anterograde amnesia; minimal depressant effect on cardiac output.
- **Side-effects**:
  - confusion;
  - unpredictable when used in the elderly.
- **Points to note**:
  - benzodiazepines consist of a benzene ring, a diazepine ring and a third ring which differentiates between the drugs.

INHALED ANAESTHETICS

Isoflurane

- **Mode of action**: global cortical depression – many receptors involved.
- **Speed of induction**: 2–3 minutes; not often used as an induction agent as it makes people cough.
- **Concentration for induction**: 5%.
- **Concentration for maintenance**: 1–1.5%.
- **Colour code**: purple.
- **Minimum alveolar concentration (MAC) value** (see Chapter 8, In the operating theatre): 1.3 in inhaled oxygen, 0.6 in nitrous oxide.
- **Advantages**:
  - concentrations up to a MAC of 1 do not increase cerebral/coronary blood flow so it is popular in neurosurgery and cardiac surgery.

- **Side-effects**:
  - hypotension and tachycardia;
  - respiratory depression;
  - pungent smell.
- **Points to note**:
  - used for maintenance as pungent odour prevents use as an inducer;
  - no analgesic properties.

Sevoflurane

- **Mode of action**: as for isoflurane. Halogenated hydrocarbon with a low boiling point; therefore, it vaporizes at ambient temperatures and is subsequently inhaled by the patient. It has a low solubility, which means there are quick changes in anaesthetic depth.
- **Speed of induction**: 2–3 minutes.
- **Concentration for induction**: 6–7%.
- **Concentration for maintenance**: 2–3%.
- **Colour code**: yellow.
- **MAC value**: 2.2 in inhaled oxygen, 1.2 in nitrous oxide.
- **Advantages**:
  - smooth onset of anaesthesia with no increase in cerebral blood flow or intra-cranial pressure below MAC of 1; does not cause tachycardia.
- **Side-effects**:
  - vasodilatation;
  - hypotension (to a lesser extent than isoflurane);
  - respiratory depression.
- **Points to note**:
  - used for induction as the least unpleasant odour.

MICRO-print

Depth of anaesthesia is directly related to the tension of the anaesthetic agent in the brain.

- The barrier that the alveolar epithelium creates to diffusion into the blood is so small that the partial pressure of the agent in the alveoli is equivalent to that in the blood and therefore determines the depth of anaesthesia.
- The partial pressure of anaesthetics in the alveoli (and therefore the depth of anaesthesia) is influenced by:
  - pulmonary ventilation;
  - cardiac output;
  - solubility of the drug in the blood.

Note that the rate of onset of action is mainly determined by solubility of the agent in the blood.

7.2 MUSCLE RELAXANTS: NEUROMUSCULAR BLOCKERS

Muscle relaxants cause paralysis of all voluntary muscles. Notably this includes muscles of respiration. Therefore, a patient must be unconscious before their administration and be ventilated afterwards as spontaneous breathing is prevented.

Neuromuscular blockers are used in two main circumstances:

- when the patient is going to be intubated and ventilated;
- to facilitate the surgery, i.e. abdominal surgery.

There are two classes of muscle relaxants.

NON-COMPETITIVE/DEPOLARIZING NEUROMUSCULAR BLOCKING DRUGS

Suxamethonium

- **Mode of action**: causes prolonged depolarization of the muscle membrane on the motor end plate by blocking receptors, meaning acetylcholine is unable to initiate muscle contraction.
- **Clinical effects**: initial contraction of the muscle, causing fasciculations lasting a few seconds, then paralysis, which lasts up to 5 minutes.
- **Onset of action**: faster than competitive muscle relaxants.
- **Indications for use**:
  - rapid sequence inductions: owing to the fast onset of action can intubate very quickly after induction of anaesthesia to prevent regurgitation of stomach contents;
  - when the patient is to be intubated but subsequently allowed to breathe spontaneously, i.e. ear, nose and throat surgery.
- **Side-effects**:
  - severe muscle pains post-operatively;
  - bradycardia;
  - raised intra-ocular pressure;
  - rise in plasma potassium.

COMPETITIVE/NON-DEPOLARIZING NEUROMUSCULAR BLOCKING DRUGS

Atracurium

- **Mode of action**: competitive antagonism of acetylcholine at the neuromuscular junction.
- **Duration of action**: 15–20 minutes. Therefore, given in repeated increments or in an infusion for prolonged procedures. Doses can be titrated accurately by the use of peripheral nerve stimulators.

Practice of anaesthesia

- **Time to intubation**: 90–120 seconds.
- **Advantages**: no effect on other body systems.
- **Elimination**: spontaneous deacetylation and hepatic metabolism.
- **Side-effects**:
  - in general, few side-effects:
    - elongated effect in hepatic failure;
    - histamine release.
- **Points to note**:
  - owing to the hepatic nature of the metabolism any enzyme inducers will speed up metabolism, e.g. phenytoin.

MICRO-print
Factors affecting a neuromuscular blockade

- Muscle blood supply. High blood flow to the muscles means early onset and short duration of action.
- Changes in temperature.
- pH.
- Potassium concentration.
- Aminoglycoside antibiotics prolong competitive blockade by reducing acetylcholine release.
- Drugs that produce central muscle relaxation, e.g. benzodiazepines/ isoflurane, prolong muscle paralysis.
- Renal disease: some competitive blockers are excreted by the kidney (e.g. rocuronium).
- Hereditary atypical cholinesterase prolongs the effect of suxamethonium, producing **suxamethonium apnoea**:
  - Cholinesterase breaks down suxamethonium.
  - In hereditary atypical cholinesterase, patients have abnormal cholinesterase, meaning that suxamethonium is broken down more slowly.
  - This leads to a prolonged duration of action of suxamethonium, which may be as long as 24 hours.
  - The drug can still be administered in these patients, but arrangements must be made for prolonged mechanical ventilation and sedation, i.e. intensive therapy unit.
  - As the condition is hereditary, families should be screened.

7.3 ANTI-CHOLINESTERASES

Anti-cholinesterases are used to reverse the paralysis of competitive muscle relaxants and allow the patient to spontaneously breathe at the end of surgery.

Anti-cholinesterases used to reverse NMB → competitive [handwritten annotation]

Anti-cholinesterases can be used in cases where neuromuscular blockers (NMBs) need to be reversed to prevent lengthy ventilation after surgery has finished. However, short-acting NMBs can be used and the last dose timed with the end of the operation to avoid using anti-cholinesterases.

NEOSTIGMINE

- **Mode of action**: principally to increase the agonist at the neuromuscular junction. In this case the agonist is acetylcholine. It is too dangerous to give acetylcholine directly and therefore the breakdown of the agonist is prevented by giving anti-cholinesterase. This increases the amount of acetylcholine, meaning it can compete for receptors on the muscle end plate and exert its effect.
- **Speed of action**: 5 minutes.
- **Duration of action**: 20–30 minutes.
- **Side-effects**:
  - Acetylcholine levels, and therefore its effects, are increased all over the body, not just at the nicotinic receptors on the neuromuscular junction but also at the muscarinic receptors in the parasympathetic nervous system. Therefore, its use causes parasympathetic side-effects such as:
    - bradycardia, decreased cardiac output;
    - spasm of the bowel;
    - nausea and vomiting;
    - bronchoconstriction;
    - miosis and blurred vision.
  - Parasympathetic effects are decreased by giving an anti-muscarinic drug, i.e. atropine or glycopyrrolate, at the same time.
- **Elimination**: it is hydrolysed by acetylcholinesterase and by plasma cholinesterase. There is also some hepatic activity.
- **Advantages**: good duration of action; does not cross the blood–brain barrier.

7.4 LOCAL ANAESTHETICS

Local anaesthetics block neuronal transmission directly; they can be administered topically, subcutaneously or adjacent to nerves. There are two forms of local anaesthetic: esters and amides. Esters are less commonly used than amides. Esters are mainly used topically as they cause more toxicity and allergic reactions.

MODE OF ACTION   *Block sodium channel* [handwritten annotation]

- Local anaesthetics work by blocking sodium channels, which means that an action potential cannot be generated, and thus the transmission of pain signals is reduced.
- The drugs exist in either ionized or non-ionized forms (weak bases).

Practice of anaesthesia

- The drug will be ionized in solution at pH 6.0. After injection the pH becomes 7.4 and the drug becomes un-ionized and can be transported into the cell.
- Intra-cellularly the pH is lower again at 7.1; this recreates the ionized form, which is then attracted to the sodium channels.
- The amount of the drug that is un-ionized will therefore increase the speed of action, but the amount that is ionized will affect the amount that is active.
- This is affected by pH of tissues and by the pKa of the drug, with a higher pKa giving higher ionization.
- The duration of action will be affected by:
  - the amount of drug that is protein bound (i.e. membrane proteins);
  - blood flow in the area, which will affect removal of the drug.
- The anaesthesia starts by blocking unmyelinated nerves, followed by myelinated ones, which gives a sequence of:
  - vasodilatation (autonomic);
  - pain;
  - loss of touch sensation;
  - paralysis (motor).

CLINICAL EFFECTS

Central nervous system

- The central nervous system (CNS) is only affected when there is toxicity due to excess systemic distribution. Typical effects with increasing severity are:
  - numbness of mouth and lips (circumoral);
  - metallic taste;
  - lightheadedness;
  - slurred speech;
  - muscle twitching;
  - convulsions.

Cardiovascular system

- Most local anaesthetics cause vasodilatation both locally via direct action and systemically via sympathetic blockade. Cocaine is an important exception, and is used in ENT surgery to prevent excessive bleeding.
- With increasing levels of drug there is initially excitability manifested by tachycardia and hypertension. This is followed by suppression manifested by hypotension, bradycardia and arrhythmias, and can lead to a cardiac arrest.

Respiratory system

- Bronchodilatation can be seen.
- If there is central toxicity apnoea can occur.

ESTER-LINKED AGENTS

Amethocaine

Only available as a gel for topical anaesthesia; usually used in children for venepuncture or cannulation.

- **Speed of action**: 45 minutes.
- **Duration of action**: 4–6 hours.
- **Side-effects**: should not be applied to damaged skin or mucosal surfaces.
- **Elimination**: hydrolysis by plasma cholinesterase.

Cocaine

Is usually used in ENT surgery as its vasoconstrictive properties mean that it reduces blood loss. It is available in solution and pastes.

- **Speed of action**: rapid.
- **Duration of action**: 20–30 minutes.
- **Side-effects** (if administered systemically):
    - **CNS**: euphoria, hyperthermia, altered vision, decreased sleep, agitation, psychosis, paranoia and suicidal tendency.
    - **Cardiovascular system**: tachycardia and arrythmias.
    - **Respiratory system**: depression of respiration.
- **Elimination**:
    - detoxified in the liver or excreted by the kidneys (10%); one breakdown product is a CNS stimulant (ecognine).

AMINE-LINKED AGENTS

Bupivacaine

- **Speed of action**: nerve block 40 minutes; epidurally 15–20 minutes; intrathecally 30 seconds.
- **Duration of action**: nerve block up to 24 hours; epidurally 3–4 hours; intrathecally 2–3 hours.
- **Side-effects**: more prone to causing cardiac toxicity than other local anaesthetic agents.
- **Elimination**: by N-dealkylation to pipecolyoxylidine and other metabolites; these are excreted in the urine.

MICRO-facts

Bupivacaine is commonly used for spinal anaesthesia. Using plain bupivacaine allows spread upwards as well as down, which can cause a rising blockade endangering respiratory function. If dextrose is added, then it becomes 'heavy' and will flow more predictably down the spine, only affecting non-essential nerves. Plain solution causes less hypotension, but the patient must be lying down.

Practice of anaesthesia

Lidocaine

- **Speed of onset**: rapid.
- **Maximum dose**: 3–5 mg/kg.
- **Duration of action**: short; 60–180 minutes depending on usage.
- **Side-effects**: cardiac toxicity is lower than that of bupivacaine.
- **Metabolism**:
  - in the liver; *N*-dealkylation followed by hydrolysis to produce metabolites that are excreted in the urine.

MICRO-facts

Lidocaine is a very popular local anaesthetic and is used for nerve blocks, infiltration and intravenous regional anaesthesia, as well as topically, epidurally and intrathecally. However, it is also a class 1B anti-arrhythmic and can be used in the treatment of tachycardias.

Prilocaine

1. **Speed of onset**: similar to lidocaine.
2. **Duration of action**: similar to lidocaine.
3. **Side-effects**: when given in doses above 600 mg, it can cause methaemoglobinaemia. This can cause cyanosis and a shift of the oxygen dissociation curve, preventing oxygen liberation at the tissue level (methylene blue reverses the process).
4. **Elimination**:
   - prilocaine is metabolized to *o*-toluidine in the lungs, liver and kidneys. This is then broken down to hydroxytoluidine.

Ropivacaine

- **Speed of onset**: similar to bupivacaine.
- **Duration of action**: shorter than bupivacaine.
- **Side-effects**: half as cardiotoxic as bupivacaine.
- **Elimination**:
  - undergoes aromatic hydroxylation to 3-hydroxyropivacaine and *N*-dealkylation; these products are mainly excreted in the urine.

MICRO-facts

The lower lipid solubility of ropivacaine means that, at lower doses, C fibres (sensory) are more preferentially blocked than A fibres (motor). This means that motor function can be spared or recover quicker while achieving a satisfactory sensory blockade.

Adrenaline

- Commonly added to local anaesthestics to be used as a vasoconstrictor. This has positive benefits in that it reduces systemic absorption.
- It reduces toxicity and extends the duration of action.
- It is most commonly used in infiltrative and nerve block techniques rather than epidurally and intrathecally.
- Its side-effects, if used around extremities, can cause necrosis owing to a lack of collateral circulation.

In the operating theatre

8.1 DELIVERING ANAESTHESIA

GASES IN THE OPERATING THEATRE

- Most hospitals use a piped system of gas and vacuum delivery to operating theatres.
- Gas cylinders are used as a back-up for pipe failures.
- The pipe system consists of colour-coded wall-mounted outlets which supply the anaesthetic machine via a flexible hose.
- The components are:
  - oxygen (white);
  - nitrous oxide (blue);
  - air (black and white);
  - vacuum (yellow).

For further information, see: http://www.boconline.co.uk/pdf_downloads/health_and_safety/gas_safety/healthcare_cylinder_id_chart.pdf

Oxygen

- Gaseous oxygen is delivered from a central liquid oxygen reserve kept cold and under pressure ($-180°C$ and 1200 kPa).
- The hotter, gaseous layer is siphoned off leaving the cooled liquid.

Nitrous oxide

- Nitrous oxide (N_2O) is delivered to theatres from cylinders kept at room temperature and under pressure as a liquid.
- N_2O has a minimum alveolar concentration (MAC) (see pp. 110–11) of over 100, so it would only be possible to adequately anaesthetize someone with N_2O using a hyperbaric chamber.
- In practice, N_2O can be used in the vaporized anaesthetic gas mixture to reduce the amount of other anaesthetic agents required.

Medical air

- Medical air has been dried, filtered and warmed before it reaches theatres via a compressor or in cylinders.

- Medical air is used both for the ventilation systems (at low pressure) and for surgical equipment requiring power (at high pressure).

Vacuum

- The vacuum consists of lengths of flexible piping connected to pumps able to exert a vacuum of at least 400 mmHg below atmospheric pressure.
- This is used for suction during surgery and contamination is avoided by the addition of filters and drains between the pump and outlets.

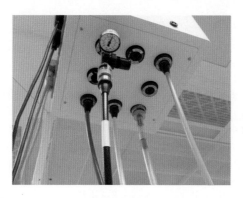

Fig. 8.1 Gas delivery.

THE ANAESTHETIC MACHINE

The modern anaesthetic machine combines:

- a gas management system;
- a breathing system;
- a way to mechanically ventilate the patient;
- a monitoring system.

Gas management system

- **Reduces pressure**:
  - Pressure from the gas source is high and needs to be lowered before being delivered to the patient.
  - This is achieved by passing the gas through a series of pressure-reducing valves, reducing pressures from ~400 kPa to ~140 kPa.
- **Controls the flow rate of gases to the patient**:
  - The flow of gases is controlled via **flowmeters**.
  - Older machines use **rotameters**, similar to that of bedside oxygen sources.
  - Calibration is essential for different gases, as both viscosity and density affect turbulence through the casing.

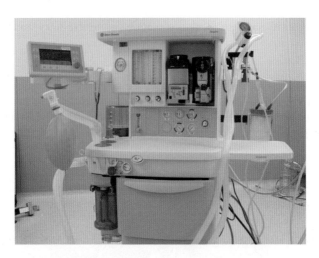

Fig. 8.2 Anaesthetic machine.

- Modern anaesthetic machines have replaced rotameters with **solenoid valve flow controllers**, which allow greater accuracy and a more complex integrated electronically managed system.
- **Adds anaesthetic vapours to gases for delivery**:
  - Volatile anaesthetic vapours are added to the gases inhaled by the patient during surgery by **vaporisers**. Classically, this is done by a **plenum vaporiser**. Modern machines simply inject liquid vapour into the gas stream, controlled by solenoids.

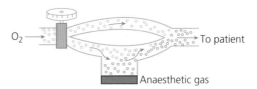

Fig. 8.3 Plenum vaporiser.

- The plenum vaporiser allows some of the gas entering it to pass through the vaporisation chamber while the rest is forced around it.
- The emerging product has a carrier gas content (the original, unchanged gas that entered) and anaesthetic vapour.
- This process allows an exact ratio of carrier gas to vapour to be created, called the **splitting ratio**.

- Vaporisers must be kept at a **constant temperature** to ensure that the volatile gases remain gas and are not converted to liquid as a result of cooling:
  - Bellows in the chamber reduce the flow of gas if the temperature falls.

Breathing system

Breathing systems are not to be confused with ventilators. They supply fresh gas to the patient and take away CO_2 but do not drive gases into or out of the patient.

- A mixture of gases and vapours is delivered via the airway management device used at induction (mask, laryngeal mask airway, endotracheal tube, etc.).

Types of breathing systems

- **Open systems**: simplest breathing system. Includes nasal cannulae and simple oxygen face masks.
- **Closed systems**: sealed circuits which deliver precise amounts of O_2. Split into:
  - **Rebreathing**: allows previously expired air to be rebreathed.
  - **Non-rebreathing**: prevents rebreathing by valves, CO_2 absorbers or high flow rates.
  - **Semi-closed**:
    - Semi-closed systems reuse gas from the previous breath that had ventilated dead space and left the patient relatively unchanged, but vent the rest of the gas expired, which is oxygen-depleted and CO_2-rich alveolar gas.
    - These systems are efficient in patients who are independently breathing, but work poorly in ventilated patients.
  - **Circle**:
    - The circle system is more complex than the semi-closed and is able to recirculate exhaled gas.
    - It uses a unidirectional valve system, so the exhaled air is forced round a circuit; the CO_2 is absorbed and small amounts of fresh gas are added:
      - ○ This improves the machine's economy and reduces pollution. Fresh gas flow can be extremely low, which also reduces addition of anaesthetic vapours.
    - The CO_2 from exhaled gas is absorbed by a CO_2 absorber containing either soda lime or baralyme with a dye indicator to show when the crystals need replacing.

Mechanical ventilation

See Chapter 4, Airways and ventilation.

Checking the anaesthetic machine

The anaesthetic machine is complex and may appear to function normally even when faults are occurring. It must be thoroughly checked for faults prior to use in surgery. Some of the most important checks are:

- **Calibration of the oxygen analyser**:
  - **Assessing**: the oxygen analyser. It is the only anaesthetic machine monitor in low-flow anaesthesia that functions downstream of the flowmeters (unlike the fail-safe valve and the O_2 supply failure alarm) and that is, therefore, able to continuously monitor the integrity of the breathing circuit. FiO_2 is tested in the fresh gas supply in some machines.
  - **Tested by**: correct calibration prior to using the machine.

> **MICRO-reference**
> See: *Checking Anaesthetic Equipment* (London: Association of Anaes-thetists of Great Britain and Ireland, 2004; http://www.aagbi.org/sites/default/files/checking04.pdf) for a comprehensive list of checks to be made on the anaesthetic machine.

- **Low-pressure circuit leak test**:
  - **Assessing**: the flowmeter valves and gas outlets for leakages as these places are the most common sources of damage from wear and tear. Failures in these components can lead to hypoxia and/or patient awareness during surgery.
  - **Tested by**: flushing O_2 through the system. Particular systems can vary enormously in internal design, so there is not a universally approved test for leakages.
- **Circle system test**:
  - **Assessing**: the breathing system for leaks and valve incompetencies.
  - **Tested by**: pressurizing the system with oxygen and monitoring the pressure gauge.

Safety features

- **Monitoring of O_2 supply**:
  - A warning alarm will sound if the O_2 supply is compromised (i.e. by a lack of supply pressure).
  - The alarm is connected to an O_2 analyser, which measures the O_2 concentration being delivered to the patient, preventing delivery of a hypoxic mixture.

- **Oxygen bypass circuit**:
    - Allows emergency administration of O_2 to the patient, bypassing the usual route. This is controlled by indented push buttons (to prevent accidental pressing) near the gas outlet.
- **Pressure regulators**:
    - Changes in pressure caused by pipeline pressure changes or altered gas demand by the patient are evened out by regulators within the machine.

8.2 INTRA-OPERATIVE MONITORING

There are several ways in which a patient should be monitored during anaesthesia.

MICRO-facts

It is possible to get CO_2 readings from an endotracheal tube in the stomach if the patient has drunk a fizzy drink immediately prior to induction.

PULSE OXIMETRY

- See Chapter 5, Oxygen.

CAPNOGRAPHY

- Measurement of end-expiration CO_2 is directly correlated with the concentration of CO_2 in arterial blood.
- Capnography is used:
    - for assessment of alveolar ventilation success;
    - for maintenance of normocapnia during mechanical ventilation;
    - for demonstrating breathing equipment is connected properly;
    - for demonstrating that the endotracheal tube is in the trachea and not the oesophagus;
    - to provide initial signs of malignant hyperthermia;
    - to indicate decreased cardiac output in a patient with a normal breathing rate (e.g. pulmonary embolism, cardiac arrest or severe hypovolaemia). This manifests itself as a gradually decreasing CO_2 level, as less CO_2 reaches the lungs from the circulation leading to a ventilation–perfusion mismatch.
- Alarms can be set to warn when CO_2 levels drop to dangerous limits.

Practice of anaesthesia

ECG

- The ECG monitors the heart rate and rhythm. This is important as it shows:
    - ischaemia;
    - electrolyte disturbance;
    - heart block;
    - cardiac arrest.
- Three-lead ECG is often used, giving a tracing equivalent to the rhythm strip of a 12-lead ECG (lead II).

MICRO-facts

A way to remember the position of these three leads:

Red = **R**ight shoulder
Ye**L**low = **L**eft shoulder
Green = Spl**een** (lower left side of the chest)

BLOOD PRESSURE (NON-INVASIVE)

- Blood pressure (BP) is continually assessed using a BP cuff to estimate end-organ perfusion.
- Automated BP systems are commonly used during anaesthesia.
- These provide the anaesthetist with three readings:
    - **systolic pressure**: fluctuations in arterial pulsation indicate the systolic BP;
    - **mean arterial pressure (MAP)**: derived from the peak pulsation amplitude, giving the most accurate of the three readings;
    - **diastolic pressure**: calculated by the machine, using an algorithm, and is therefore the least accurate reading.
- A systolic pressure of <90 mmHg could be indicative of inadequate end-organ perfusion, although this is highly patient dependent.
- The frequency of repeat measurements can be chosen as required.

BLOOD PRESSURE (INVASIVE)

- Indications:
    - cardiovascular compromise;
    - use of inotropes/vasodilators;

- obesity (rendering non-invasive measures inaccurate).
- BP is assessed by inserting an arterial line peripherally.
- **Advantages**: continuous and immediate monitoring.
- **Disadvantages**: occasionally a difficult procedure. Displacement of line causing haemorrhage.
- **Sources of error**: clots, air emboli.

TEMPERATURE

- **Anaesthetics affect temperature homeostasis**. Therefore patients are at risk of temperature fluctuations during anaesthesia.
- Many agents increase the sweating threshold while decreasing the shivering and vasoconstriction threshold, and also redistribute heat from the core to the peripheries.
- Core (oral, axillary, rectal or bladder temperatures), rather than tympanic, temperature must be monitored. Tympanic temperature is highly unreliable owing to waxy build-up in the canal giving misleading results.
- Temperature is extremely important to monitor:
  - malignant hyperthermia can become clinically evident by a rapidly increasing temperature;
  - core hypothermia is life-threatening. It can occur in both general and regional techniques.
- An intra-operative core temperature should ideally be maintained at above 36°C, unless hypothermia is being used to prevent cerebral ischaemia (e.g. during cardiac surgery).

DEPTH OF ANAESTHESIA

- Depth of anaesthesia must be assessed during the induction and maintenance.
- Plasma concentration of the induction agent will peak and decrease within minutes, causing a fluctuation.
- Signs of adequate depth of anaesthesia in the induction include:
  - loss of verbal responses and eyelid and corneal reflexes;
  - an increase in heart rate and BP during noxious stimulation, such as laryngoscopy and intubation, is rarely completely eradicated by the intravenous (IV) induction agent.
- Inadequate maintenance anaesthesia can be shown by:
  - systemic arterial BP increase of >15 mmHg higher than the patient's usual;
  - heart rate increase to >90 beats/min in the absence of hypovolaemia;
  - muscle movement;
  - autonomic signs such as lacrimation, skin flushing or sweating.

Practice of anaesthesia

- The depth of anaesthesia can be quickly corrected by increasing the dose of anaesthetic agent and can be indicated by the MAC value.

MICRO-facts

Maintenance anaesthesia can be extremely difficult to gauge. For example, increased blood pressure and heart rate could be signs of inadequate analgesia rather than inadequate anaesthesia.

CENTRAL VENOUS PRESSURE

See above under Blood pressure (invasive).
- The central venous pressure (CVP) is used to give a more accurate representation of volume status than the pressure cuff.
- Generally, patients requiring a CVP measurement will be those undergoing:
    - long operations in which fluid shift can be expected;
    - operations in which significant blood loss can be expected;
    - small operations in patients who are ill-equipped to deal with any fluid shift (e.g. heart failure).
- A low CVP indicates hypovolaemia and requires a fluid challenge (a truly hypovolaemic patient will respond initially and then go back to a low CVP, whereas a euvolaemic patient will have a CVP which continues to increase).

MICRO-print
Central venous pressure will be affected by many things:
- patient posture/table positioning;
- fluid status;
- heart failure;
- increased intra-thoracic pressure (e.g. intermittent positive pressure ventilation);
- pulmonary embolism;
- pulmonary hypertension;
- valvular disease;
- pericardial effusion;
- superior vena cava obstruction.

BLOOD LOSS

- Blood loss must be monitored to ensure correct fluid management.
- This can be assessed by:
    - Weighing soaked swabs used in the operation.

- Measuring the volume of blood in the suction container:
  - washing and analysing the resultant solute for blood (mainly used in children).
- Blood gas and pH analysis (often performed during cardiac bypass).
- Clotting studies and haemoglobin concentration of patients receiving blood products.
- However, blood loss is difficult to accurately determine, so the anaesthetist must continually assess clinically.

PERIPHERAL NERVE STIMULATOR

- Peripheral nerve stimulators are used:
  - when administering a neuromuscular blocking drug;
  - to assess whether there is residual neuromuscular blockade after surgery.
- Nerve stimulators pass an electrical impulse from the transmitter to a nerve via surface electrodes.
- Watching or feeling for contraction or measuring the force or action potential allows assessment of nerve transmission.

MINIMUM ALVEOLAR CONCENTRATION

- **MAC**:
  - The concentration of anaesthetic vapour within the alveoli which will prevent movement in response to a skin cut in 50% of the population at 1 atmosphere.

MICRO-reference

For further information, see: http://www.anesthesia-analgesia.org/content/93/4/947.full

---

MICRO-print

Minimum alveolar concentration values are measured in percentage volumes of an anaesthetic.

Practical uses of MAC

- MAC values are used to indicate the potency of an inhalational anaesthetic agent.
- Most inhaled agents have a different MAC value.
- The MAC value which registers on the anaesthetic machine is used as a guideline to titrate the concentration of anaesthetic agent delivered to the patient.
- There are several factors which may affect MAC values and which do not show on the machine (Table 8.1).

Practice of anaesthesia

Table 8.1 Factors affecting minimum alveolar concentration (MAC)

REDUCES MAC	INCREASES MAC
Increasing age	Decreasing age
Sedatives and analgesics	Adrenaline or amphetamines
Nitrous oxide	Thyrotoxicosis
Drugs which affect neurotransmitter release	Chronic alcoholism
Higher atmospheric pressure	Pyrexia
Hypotension	
Hypothermia	
Pregnancy	

8.3 INTRA-OPERATIVE EMERGENCIES AND COMPLICATIONS

ASPIRATION OF GASTRIC CONTENTS

- **Signs suggestive of aspiration**:
  - Coughing during induction.
  - Gastric contents in the pharynx at laryngoscopy, or around the edge of the face mask.
  - Hypoxia.
  - Bronchospasm.
- **Management**:
  - Maintain airway.
  - Position bed head down, with the patient on his or her left side.
  - Aspirate material from the pharynx under **direct vision** using a laryngoscope.
  - If neuromuscular blockers have not been given and the surgery is not essential:
    - 100% oxygen, cricoid pressure and ventilate if not breathing;
    - allow the patient to recover from anaesthesia;
    - salbutamol ± ipratropium to treat bronchospasm;
    - chest radiograph;
    - high-dependency unit (HDU)/intensive therapy unit (ITU) care.
  - If neuromuscular blockers not given but the surgery is essential:
    - nasogastric tube to empty the stomach;
    - allow the patient to recover from general anaesthesia;
    - perform a rapid sequence induction and continue surgery;

- – aspirate the tracheobronchial tree;
- – salbutamol $\pm$ ipratropium to treat bronchospasm;
- – chest radiograph;
- – HDU/ITU care.
- If neuromuscular blockers have been given:
  - – rapid sequence induction;
  - – aspirate the tracheobronchial tree;
  - – start positive pressure ventilation;
  - – bronchopulmonary lavage with saline;
  - – salbutamol $\pm$ ipratropium to treat bronchospasm;
  - – nasogastric tube to empty stomach.

ANAPHYLAXIS

> ### MICRO-facts
>
> **Anaphylaxis:** a severe, life-threatening generalized hypersensitivity reaction affecting cardiopulmonary function.

- **Signs suggestive of anaphylaxis**:
  - Hypotension.
  - Bronchospasm.
  - Flushing.
  - Hypoxaemia.
  - Urticaria.
  - Angioedema.
  - Pruritus.
  - Nausea and vomiting.
- **Common causes of anaphylaxis**:
  - Anaesthetic agents.
  - Muscle relaxants.
  - Induction agents.
  - Antibiotics, e.g. penicillin.
  - IV fluids, e.g. colloids.
  - Other, e.g. latex.

> ### MICRO-reference
> For management of anaphylaxis in the context of anaesthesia, see:
> http://www.aagbi.org/sites/default/files/anaphylaxis_2009.pdf

Practice of anaesthesia

> ## MICRO-facts
> Do NOT ever use IV adrenaline unless trained to do so.

- **Management**:
  - ABC approach.
  - **Stop all likely precipitants**.
  - Elevate patient's legs (if hypotensive).
  - **Adrenaline**:
    - initial dose of 0.5 mL of 1:10 000 intravenously. Several doses might be required and an infusion can be started if necessary.
  - Ventilation: airway must be secured if spontaneous ventilation is inadequate $\pm$ bronchospasm. Either intubate or use a surgical airway.
  - Circulatory support: fast IV saline.
  - Monitoring: ECG, saturations, BP, end-tidal CO_2, CVP, urine output.
  - Anti-histamines: chlorpheniramine.
  - Steroids: hydrocortisone.
  - Bronchodilators: salbutamol.
  - HDU/ITU care: monitor for biphasic reaction.
  - Plasma tryptase: blood samples taken immediately after treatment, then 1–2 hours after the event and a third sample 24 hours after the event. Elevation of plasma tryptase confirms that the reaction was associated with mast cell degranulation (and in doing so confirms anaphylaxis).

MALIGNANT HYPERTHERMIA

> ## MICRO-facts
> **Malignant hyperthermia:** rare inherited disorder of skeletal muscle metabolism triggered by exposure to inhaled anaesthetic agents and suxamethonium, in which there is release of abnormally high concentrations of calcium from the sarcoplasmic reticulum causing increased muscle metabolism. This leads to excess heat production causing a rise in core temperature of at least 2°C/h.

> ### MICRO-reference
> For diagnosis and management, see:
> http://www.aagbi.org/sites/default/files/malignanthyp07amended_0.pdf

- **Signs suggestive of malignant hyperthermia**:
  - Increased end-tidal CO_2 for no other reason (early sign).
  - Tachycardia for no other reason.
  - Tachypnoea.
  - Muscle rigidity, masseter spasm.
  - Cardiac arrythmias.
  - Falling saturations and cyanosis.
  - Rise in temperature of $2°C/h$ (a late sign).
- **Management**:
  - Stop all anaesthetic agents.
  - Use a clean breathing circuit with high-flow, non-rebreathe oxygen.
  - Use IV agents such as propofol for maintenance until surgery finished.
  - Monitor temperature.
  - Dantrolene: inhibits calcium release, preventing further muscle activity.
  - Active cooling:
    - cold normal saline IV;
    - expose the patient completely;
    - ice over axillary and femoral arteries;
    - fanning;
    - gastric/peritoneal lavage with cold normal saline.
  - Monitor for complications:
    - acidosis;
    - hyperkalaemia;
    - renal failure;
    - coagulopathy.
  - Correct acidosis and hypoxaemia with bicarbonate and hyperventilation.
  - Treat hyperkalaemia, myoglobinaemia, disseminated intravascular coagulation and cardiac arrhythmias.
- Screen patient's family for susceptibility to malignant hyperthermia.

HYPOTENSION

MICRO-facts

Hypotension: an abnormally low blood pressure (BP). There are no absolute values as they vary from patient to patient, although systolic BP < 100 mmHg with diastolic BP < 40 mmHg is often considered abnormally low. It is important to consider the patient's usual resting BP – are they usually hypertensive? If so, the threshold for considering hypotension may be a higher BP. Often determined using mean arterial pressure (MAP), in which hypotension is a 25% reduction in MAP.

Practice of anaesthesia

- **Problems arising from hypotension**:
  - Poor tissue perfusion leading to acidaemia.
  - Acute kidney injury (see later under Acute kidney injury).
  - Decreased cerebral perfusion pressure (CPP):
    - important particularly in neurosurgical operations;
    - **CPP = MAP − ICP**, where ICP is intra-cranial pressure;
    - MAP is kept >80 in suspected raised ICP.
  - Cerebrovascular accident.
  - Myocardial infarction.
  - Fetal compromise (in obstetric patients).
- **Signs suggestive of poor tissue perfusion**:
  - Fall in BP.
  - Dizziness, nausea and vomiting (in regional anaesthesia).
  - Confusion (poor cerebral perfusion).
  - Fall in urine output (poor renal perfusion).
  - Rhythm changes, ST elevation.
- **Risk factors for developing intra-operative hypotension**:
  - Hypertension and peripheral vascular disease.
  - Cardiovascular disease (especially those causing fixed cardiac output).
  - Hypovolaemia (sepsis, extensive blood loss from surgery, burns, vomiting, etc.).
  - Combined regional and general anaesthesia.
- **Management**:
  - Use ABC approach.
  - If severe, call for assistance.
  - Consider cause.
  - Reduce anaesthetic (avoiding awareness).
  - Optimize pre-load: fluid challenge, elevate legs.
  - Increase contractility: positive inotrope (e.g. ephedrine).
  - Counteract systemic vasodilatation: systemic vasoconstrictor (e.g. phenylephrine, metaraminol, ephedrine).

ACUTE KIDNEY INJURY

MICRO-facts

Acute kidney injury (AKI): an **abrupt, sustained decline** in renal function. The **RIFLE** criteria are used to grade AKI: **R**isk, **I**njury, **F**ailure, **L**oss and **E**nd-stage kidney disease. Hypoperfusion can lead to pre-renal azotaemia, which results in an ischaemic insult to the kidneys. This causes acute tubular necrosis and acute renal dysfunction or failure.

- **Signs suggestive of acute kidney injury**:
  - Decreased urine output.
- **Risk factors for developing acute kidney injury**:
  - Patient factors:
    - dehydration and hypovolaemia (often secondary to illness);
    - pre-existing renal dysfunction;
    - diabetes;
    - sepsis;
    - jaundice/liver failure;
    - cardiac dysfunction;
    - nephrotoxic drugs: these include certain antibiotics, anti-hypertensives, non-steroidal anti-inflammatory drugs, furosemide, immunosuppressives and radiological contrast media.
  - **Anaesthetic factors**:
    - prolonged hypotension;
    - inadequate hydration;
    - note that these are both commonly peri-operative problems, as anaesthetic time is usually short.
  - **Surgical factors**:
    - cardiopulmonary bypass;
    - aortic cross-clamping;
    - renal/liver transplant;
    - abdominal compartment syndrome.
- **Management**:
  - Optimize fluid treatment and blood pressure.
  - Treat sepsis if present.
  - Stop nephrotoxic agents if possible.
  - Haemofiltration.
  - HDU/ITU referral.

Practice of anaesthesia

Part III

On the wards

9 Post-operative complications

- The highest rates of morbidity and mortality occur in the post-operative period.
- Most complications occur 1–3 days after the operation.

9.1 COMMON COMPLICATIONS

IMMEDIATE

- Pain.
- Bleeding.
- **Shock** (Table 9.1):
    - hypovolaemic (acute blood loss);
    - cardiogenic (acute myocardial infarction/pulmonary embolism);
    - septic;
    - anaphylactic;
    - neurogenic (spinal or general anaesthesia).
- Basal atelectasis.
- Low urine output.

EARLY

- Pain.
- Post-operative nausea and vomiting (PONV).
- **Shock** (Table 9.1).
- Acute confusion.
- Cardiac events.
- **Infection**:
    - pneumonia;
    - urinary tract infection;
    - wound infection.
- Wound/anastomosis dehiscence.
- Deep vein thrombosis (DVT)/pulmonary embolism (PE).
- Acute urinary retention.
- Paralytic ileus.

Table 9.1 Types of shock

	DECREASED PRE-LOAD PERIPHERAL CIRCULATION FAILURE	DECREASED CONTRACTILITY PUMP FAILURE	DECREASED AFTERLOAD PERIPHERAL CIRCULATION FAILURE
Signs	Low JVP Postural hypotension Cool skin/clammy	High JVP/CVP Cool skin/clammy Pulmonary oedema	Low JVP Bounding pulse Warm skin
Problem	Hypovolaemic	Failure of the heart to maintain circulation	Distributive
Type of shock	Hypovolaemic shock	Cardiogenic shock	Septic shock Anaphylactic shock Neurogenic shock

Causes	Inadequate fluid intake
	  Dehydration
	External fluid loss
	  Vomiting
	  Diarrhoea
	  Haemorrhage
	  Polyuria
	Internal fluid loss
	  Burns
	  Third space sequestration
	  High-output fistula
		ACS
		Arrhythmia
		Tamponade
		Myocarditis
		PE
		Tension pneumothorax
		Aortic dissection
			See Decreased pre-load

ACS, acute coronary syndromes; CVP, central venous pressure; JVP, jugular venous pressure; PE, pulmonary embolism.

LATE

- Adhesion formation.
- Incisional hernia.
- Loss of mobility.
- Chronic pain.
- Failure of surgery/recurrence of original pathology.

9.2 SEPSIS

- **Systemic inflammatory response syndrome** (SIRS) – two or more of:
  - abnormal body temperature ($<36°C$ or $>38°C$);
  - raised heart rate (>90 beats/min);
  - raised respiratory rate (>20 breaths/min);
  - altered white blood cell count ($>12000/mm^3$ or $<4000/mm^3$, or $>10\%$ immature neutrophils).
- **Sepsis**: SIRS in the presence of infection.
- **Severe sepsis**: sepsis with evidence of organ dysfunction.
- **Septic shock**: severe sepsis in which the patient remains hypotensive despite administration of fluid challenges.

MORTALITY

- Severe sepsis: 30%.
- Severe sepsis in the elderly: 40%.
- Septic shock: 50%.
- Responsible for approximately 36,800 deaths per year.

PATHOPHYSIOLOGY

- Sepsis occurs as a result of an infective microbial insult.
- Various components of bacteria, fungi, viruses or parasites are detected by the host and lead to the immune system response.
- Sepsis is thought to be a result of an unbalanced response of pro- and anti-inflammatory reactions:
  - **Proinflammatory reactions**:
    - include cytokine-mediated pathology (with production of cytokines such as tumour necrosis factor α, interleukin (IL)-1 and IL-6), coagulation activation and complement activation;
    - intended to kill invading pathogens but cause tissue damage;
    - lead to early mortality and acute organ dysfunction.
  - **Anti-inflammatory responses**:
    - involve IL-4 and IL-10;
    - cause apoptosis of immune cells.
  - This disordered immune response has various adverse effects:
    - decreased vascular tone;

On the wards

- loss of tone in arterioles responsible for blood pressure (BP) regulation;
- decreased blood flow;
- decreased organ perfusion;
- loss of endothelial cell integrity;
- damage to the vascular endothelial barrier allowing leak of proteins and macromolecules; leak results in exaggerated movement of fluid across the vasculature to the extra-cellular space.
- Sepsis leads to high mortality.

MICRO-facts

The **sepsis six** are actions that must be taken within 1 hour:
1. Give high-flow oxygen (15 litres via non-rebreather mask).
2. Take blood cultures.
3. Give intravenous (IV) antibiotics.
4. Start IV fluid resuscitation.
5. Check haemoglobin and lactate.
6. Monitor accurate hourly urine output.

MANAGEMENT

MICRO-reference

For useful information of management of sepsis, see:
http://www.survivingsepsis.org/guidelines.

- ABCDE resuscitation (see Chapter 11, Recognizing and managing ill patients).
- Intravenous (IV) access.
- Bloods: full blood count (FBC), urea and electrolytes (U&Es), blood cultures.
- Arterial blood gas (ABG).
- **Early antibiotics**.

MICRO-case

Mrs P is a 68 year old woman who was admitted to hospital for a colorectal carcinoma. It is now 2 days since her operation. The surgical ward's junior doctor is asked to review her, as her early warning score has been recorded as 3 (for heart rate, blood pressure and temperature). When the junior doctor reviews her, he finds:

continued...

continued...

A: patent, maintaining her own airway.

B: respiratory rate, 21; chest clear; O_2 saturations 98% on 2 litres O_2.

C: capillary refill time, 3 seconds; pulse, 105; blood pressure (BP) 82/52 mmHg.

D: drowsy, but responsive to voice.

E: urine output has not been recorded. Abdomen is distended and tender.

The doctor decides that the current priorities are: gaining intravenous access, giving some fluid and sending off bloods.

An hour later, the surgical registrar caring for Mrs P happens to be on the ward and comes to see her. She immediately instructs the junior doctor to catheterize Mrs P, while she begins giving a fluid challenge. After giving 500 mL of normal saline, her blood pressure has gone down to 78/46 mmHg and she is less responsive. However, after 2 litres she seems to be coming round and her BP is 84/64 mmHg.

Mrs P is given high-dose antibiotics and taken straight to theatre, where it is discovered that she has an anastomotic leak with faecal peritonitis. Her abdomen is washed out and Hartmann's procedure (colostomy to allow the damaged bowel to heal before re-connecting) is performed.

Mrs P is taken to the intensive therapy unit post-operatively, where she is put on continuous venovenous haemofiltration, ventilated, given inotropic support and antibiotic treatment; 5 days later, she no longer needs multisystem support, is awake and plans are made to step-down her care and transfer her to the high dependency unit.

Points to consider:

- Early recognition and management of sepsis is key. The junior doctor should have taken note of her low blood pressure, tachycardia and delayed capillary refill time.
- A fluid challenge should be administered immediately in a patient showing signs of hypovolaemia.
- Some patients with septic shock will not respond to a fluid challenge but still require careful fluid resuscitation.
- Almost any fluid can be given in a fluid challenge, although dextrose is avoided as it rapidly moves out of vascular space into the tissues.

9.3 PAIN

- **Acute pain management**: the 'pain team'. This team of anaesthetists and specialist nurses see patients with acute pain in hospital, especially immediately post-operative patients.
- **Chronic pain management**: patients with refractory pain can be seen in specialist pain clinics.

On the wards

PHYSIOLOGY OF PAIN

- **Pain**: an unpleasant sensory and emotional experience associated with actual or potential tissue damage.

TRANSMISSION OF PAIN

> ### MICRO-facts
> **Nociceptors: free nerve endings** of **afferent** neurones that transmit pain perception via the spinothalamic tract.

- The sensation of pain is transmitted by **nociceptors** in response to actual/ assumed tissue damage of end organs.
- Nociceptors respond to:
  - mechanical deformation (from severe pressure);
  - excessive heat;
  - some chemicals;
  - neuropeptide transmitters: bradykinin, histamine, cytokines, prostaglandins (many of these substances are released from damaged cells).

> ### MICRO-print
> Referred pain occurs as a result of somatic and visceral fibres synapsing at a single interneurone. As pain signals most often originate from somatic receptors, the signal is assumed to be of somatic origin rather than visceral, and this incorrect information is passed to the brain.

Regulation of pain transmission

- All sensory information transmitted to the central nervous system (CNS) can be modulated.
- Transmission up an **afferent neurone** can be inhibited by:
  - collateral branches of other ascending neurones (known as lateral inhibition);
  - cerebral cortices via descending neurones, which can directly inhibit axons;
  - indirectly, using specific synapses.
- Regulation of pain transmission is different from the modulation of other sensory stimuli:
  - The afferent input from nociceptors is continually inhibited.

- This allows disinhibition to take place during severe tissue damage (therefore, increasing the pain signal) or complete inhibition (which would completely block the signal).
- Also, unlike other sensory transmission, changes occur in nociceptors and pain pathways after a transduction of a noxious stimulus:
  - This changes the way each part of the sensory unit will respond to further stimuli.
  - Increased pain sensation to the same stimulus is called **hyperalgesia**. This means that the pain perception caused by a stimulus will be disproportionate to the stimulus itself.
- **Allodynia** is the sensation of pain, in the absence of a painful stimulus.
- **Pain** is also **augmented** by many other sensations:
  - emotion, especially anxiety;
  - suggestion (e.g. being told something will be very painful makes it feel more painful);
  - activation of other sensory modalities (e.g. the sight of blood).

WHY PROVIDE PAIN RELIEF?

- The majority of patients in hospital will be in pain at some point and require analgesia.
- The key to successful pain management is identifying these patients early, to curb pain before the patient becomes distressed and more difficult to manage.
- All patients should be asked regularly if they are in any pain, as many – especially older patients – may not want to complain, or think nothing can be done.
- Pain relief does not just **alleviate suffering**:
  - Physiological benefits include:
    - reducing sympathetic effects of pain (tachycardia, hypertension, increased myocardial oxygen demand), which could precipitate a myocardial infarction;
    - earlier mobilization, reducing risk of DVT/PE;
    - for some operations (e.g. thoracic, upper gastrointestinal (GI)), adequate pain relief improves **post-operative survival** by allowing the patient to cough and clear secretions, reducing the risk of pneumonia, basal atelectasis, etc.;
    - reduction of chronic pain syndromes.
- Effective pain control is one of the key considerations for safe discharge.

ASSESSMENT OF PAIN SEVERITY

- **Quantification**:
  - Rating scales (from 1 to 10; no pain, mild, moderate, severe or excruciating).
  - Visual analogue scales: the patient is asked to mark the intensity of their pain on a 10 cm line.

On the wards

No pain ⌞_____⌟ Worst pain imaginable

- Functional assessment:
  - Is the patient able to mobilize with the pain?
  - Can the patient take deep breaths without pain?
  - Is the patient able to eat or drink (if appropriate).
- Biological measurements:
  - Heart rate: initial decrease and then increases.
  - Oxygen saturations: adults may desaturate, whereas children often maintain their saturation even if they have been in pain for a prolonged period.
- **Qualitative assessment**:
  - Ask the patient to describe the pain.
  - The appearance of the patient: sweating, groaning or in obvious distress; altered breathing; having difficulty or unable to move/cough.
- However the pain is assessed, it must be **rechecked regularly**. This is the only way to ensure that the patient will receive adequate analgesia.

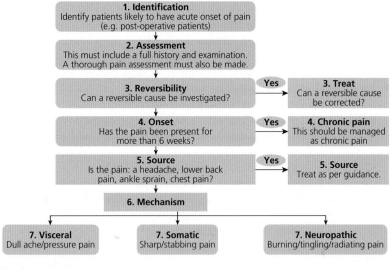

Fig. 9.1 Assessing pain.

REVERSIBILITY

- The first priority will be to treat any reversible causes of pain.

9.4 ANALGESIA

MICRO-facts

Paracetamol

- **Mechanism of action**: unknown.
- 'Simple analgesia'.
- Should be prescribed to the maximum dosage.
- Provides an effective baseline analgesia.
- Will reduce the amount of stronger analgesia needed and therefore reduce the potential side-effects. Reduce dosage in low body weight.

- Analgesia: the specific suppression of pain.
- There are two main types of systemic analgesics:
  - non-steroidal anti-inflammatory drugs (NSAIDs) and possibly paracetamol;
  - opioid analgesics.

NON-STEROIDAL ANTI-INFLAMMATORY DRUGS

- **Types**:
  - **Salicylic acid derivatives**:
    - aspirin.
  - **Propionic acid derivatives**:
    - ibuprofen;
    - naproxen.
  - **Selective cyclo-oxygenase (COX) 2 inhibitors**:
    - the -coxib family (parecoxib, etoricoxib, etc.).
  - **Others**:
    - diclofenac;
    - indometacin.
  - Broadly speaking, these drugs work by inhibiting COX enzymes (Fig. 9.2).

MICRO-facts

Nefopam is another non-opioid analgesic that does not fit into the non-steroidal category. It can be tried when other non-opioids have been unsuccesful and is widely used.

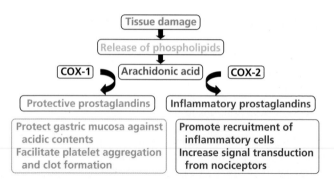

Fig. 9.2 Cyclo-oxygenase (COX) 1 and 2 pathway.

- **Traditional NSAIDs** non-selectively **inhibit COX enzymes** and are therefore associated with side-effects such as dyspepsia and gastric ulcers.
- However, some are used specifically for their inhibition of COX-1, such as aspirin.
- **COX-2 inhibitors**, such as etoricoxib, are widely used in rheumatic conditions because of their highly selective nature (COX inhibitors either selectively or non-selectively increase the risk of cardiac events).

OPIOID ANALGESICS

Pathophysiology

- Pain transmission to the CNS must go through relay neurones in the dorsal horns of the spinal cord.
- This signal can be inhibited by interneurones.
- Interneurones release **opioid peptides** such as dynorphin.
- The signal can also be inhibited by descending enkephalinergic, noradrenergic or serotonergic fibres that are activated by opioid peptides.
- The opioid peptides are mediated by **opioid receptors**.
- The main opioid receptors in the CNS are:
  - **mu (μ)**;
  - **kappa (κ)**;
  - **delta (δ)**.
- Opioid analgesics mimic opioid peptides and bind to these specific receptors.
- μ receptors are the most abundant in the CNS and are the site of action for the majority of opioid analgesics.
- **Opioid analgesics** can be either strong or weak.
  - **Strong**:
    - diamorphine;
    - morphine;
    - oxycodone;

- pentazocine;
- fentanyl;
- alfentanil;
- buprenorphine;
- pethidine.
- **Weak**:
  - codeine;
  - dihydrocodeine;
  - tramadol.

MICRO-facts

Weak opioids such as codeine are activated by metabolizing to morphine. Only around 10% is metabolized, therefore producing a much smaller response. Some people are unable to metabolize codeine, rendering it completely inactive.

PROVIDING ANALGESIA

Analgesia during surgery

- Patients are provided with analgesia during the operation, even when under general anaesthetic. This is for two reasons:
  - By reducing the response to pain during the operation, the anaesthetic can be maintained at a lower plane of anaesthesia, requiring less anaesthetic agent.
  - Additionally, intra-operative analgesia has been shown to reduce the post-operative pain reported by the patient, in particular regional analgesia.
- The World Health Organization analgesic ladder is intended for cancer pain but is applicable to all pain control.

Patient-controlled analgesia

- As pain levels experienced by different patients vary considerably over time, to give a patient analgesia more closely titrated to the levels he or she requires, patient-controlled analgesia can be used (sometimes in addition to an infusion) as part of the patient's pain management regime.
- These are devices that provide an extra 'boost' of analgesia on demand when the patient presses a button, self-administering a small bolus of analgesic.
- The opioid used in this system should have a rapid onset and moderate duration. Morphine is most commonly used.
- For safety, the parameters of bolus size, minimum time between doses (long enough to allow maximal effect of analgesic) and maximum dose (e.g. per

hour) must be carefully considered, and the patient should be educated pre-operatively about how to use the device safely and effectively.

Local anaesthesia for pain relief

- By using long-acting local anaesthetics (e.g. bupivacaine) post-surgical pain relief can last for several hours.
- With the use of catheters (e.g. epidural catheters) this benefit can be extended for days.

Transcutaneous electrical nerve stimulation

- Transcutaneous electrical nerve stimulation (TENS) involves placing electrodes in direct contact with the skin and close to the painful area. If the electrodes are placed far away then nerve stimulation is unlikely to give any analgesic benefit.
- Stimulates the large Aβ sensory fibres, aiming to cause inhibition of pain conduction.
- High-frequency, low-intensity stimulation is used to activate the fibres and is most effective when the dose of stimulation is at near-noxious levels. In practice, this should mean that patients feel a buzzing or tingling sensation on their skin.
- This level of stimulation should excite both Aβ and Aδ fibres, which produces the best level of analgesia.

REGIONAL BLOCKADE

- **Epidurals**: see Chapter 6, Local and regional anaesthesia.
- **Regional blocks**: see Chapter 6, Local and regional anaesthesia.

SPINAL BLOCKADE

See Chapter 6, Local and regional anaesthesia.

MICRO-case

A 72 year old man presents to his GP with rectal bleeding. He is referred under a 2 week wait to a colorectal surgeon, who arranges a flexible sigmoidoscopy. The patient is found to have a Dukes B rectosigmoid bowel cancer. On staging CT, this cancer is found to have no lymphatic or distant spread and he is booked for a curative high anterior resection.

The operation is successful and, on returning to the ward, he has patient controlled analgesia (PCA) *in situ*. On day 2 after the operation, the patient's use of the PCA is low and the nurse looking after him asks that you prescribe alternative analgesia so that the PCA can be taken down.

continued...

continued...

You prescribe:
Regular analgesia:
paracetamol 1 g QDS (orally or intravenous preparations);
tramadol 100 mg QDS orally.
As-required analgesia:
morphine 2.5–5 mg subcutaneously (SC) every 1–2 hours.
Remembering morphine's side-effect profile, in addition to this you also prescribe:
cyclizine 50 mg orally/intramuscularly/SC TDS.

On day 6 after the operation, the patient has not required SC morphine for 2 days. Today, however, he starts to complain of pain that is not being controlled by the medications you prescribed above. The nurse asks if there is anything else that could be tried without having to start the patient back on morphine. You prescribe nefopam.

Points to consider:

- Patients will often return from theatre with a PCA *in situ*. This should be taken down 2–3 days post-operatively, when both the patient and all members of the multidisciplinary team are happy.
- Junior doctors should use the World Health Organization's pain relief ladder as a template for prescribing analgesia.
- Tramadol is preferable to codeine phosphate in colorectal surgery as codeine phosphate can cause constipation.
- Nefopam is a non-opioid analgesic and is good for moderate pain. It is an alternative to paracetamol and compound preparations that may cause constipation.

9.5 POST-OPERATIVE NAUSEA AND VOMITING

- Post-operative nausea and vomiting (PONV) is one of the most common transient complications following surgery, affecting 20–40% of patients.
- Nausea and vomiting results in patient discomfort, anxiety, distress and morbidity.
- Vomiting increases intra-cranial and intra-ocular pressure, a problem in neurosurgical and ophthalmic patients.
- **Vomiting in a semiconscious patient can lead to loss of airway patency and to aspiration pneumonia** (see Chapter 4, Airways and ventilation).
- Effective control of PONV:
  - allows earlier discharge: if the patient is vomiting, oral drugs (antibiotics and analgesics) cannot be used;
  - reduces the chance of aspiration pneumonia.

On the wards

RISK FACTORS FOR DEVELOPING POST-OPERATIVE NAUSEA AND VOMITING

Patient risk factors

- Previous episode of PONV.
- Female.
- Age: peaks at 6–16 years.
- Anxiety.
- History of travel sickness.
- Non-smoker.

Anaesthetic risk factors

- **Drugs**:
    - opioids;
    - anaesthetic vapours (dose dependent);
    - IV induction agents (except propofol); less likely as these are usually excreted by the end of the operation;
    - nitrous oxide (affects middle ear and bowel);
    - neostigmine.
- **Techniques**:
    - gastric insufflation during intubation;
    - hypoxia;
    - subarachnoid blocks when hypotensive.

Surgical risk factors

- emergency procedures;
- duration;
- day case surgery;
- ENT, gynaecological and GI surgery;
- strabismus correction;
- high levels of post-operative pain;
- ileus;
- gastric distension (e.g. gastroscopy).

ANATOMY AND PHYSIOLOGY OF VOMITING

- The vomiting centre located in the **lateral reticular formation** of the medulla.
- **Afferent** inputs from:
    - GI tract;
    - peripheral pain receptors;
    - nucleus solitarius (gag reflex);
    - vestibular system (motion sickness);
    - cerebral cortex;

- chemoreceptor trigger zone (CTZ; in root of fourth ventricle detects circulatory drugs and toxins).
- Key neurotransmitters involved and targets for **anti-emetics** (see Chapter 2, Preparing for surgery):
  - histamine;
  - acetylcholine;
  - 5-hydroxytryptamine and dopamine (in CTZ).
- **Prevention of nausea and vomiting**:
  - give prophylactic anti-emetics whenever two or more risk factors are present;
  - consider combinations of anti-emetics if the patient is high risk for PONV;
  - consider total intravenous analgesia with propofol.

9.6 ACUTE BLOOD LOSS

Classification of blood loss is shown in Table 9.2.

- **Management**:
  - if bleeding externally, apply direct pressure to the wound.
- **Resuscitation**:
  - Insert two large-bore IV cannulas (14G; usually antecubital fossa).
  - Bloods: FBC, U&Es and cross-match.

Table 9.2 Classification of blood loss

	CLASS 1	CLASS 2	CLASS 3	CLASS 4
Blood loss (%)	< 15	15–30	30–40	> 40
Blood loss for 70 kg (mL)	750	750–1500	1500–2000	> 2000
Blood pressure	Normal	Normal	Reduced	Markedly reduced
Heart rate (beats/min)	< 100	> 100	> 120	> 140
Respiratory rate (breaths/min)	14–20	20–30	30–40	30–40
Urine output (mL/h)	> 30	20–30	10–20	< 10
Mental state	Alert	Anxious/ aggressive	Confused	Drowsy/ unconscious

- Perform ABG sampling:
  - may show marked base deficit and lactic acidosis;
  - correction suggests adequate resuscitation.
- 2 litres warm fluid appropriate for resuscitation fluid challenge, monitoring central venous pressure.
- Insert arterial cannula for BP monitoring.
- Warm fluids and monitor for hypothermia.
- If failure to improve vital signs (suggests exsanguination) or transient response to fluid challenge (suggests 20–40% blood loss):
  - Blood transfusion indicated and consider surgical input for immediate theatre:
    - ○ full cross-match takes ~45 minutes;
    - ○ group confirmed match takes ~10 minutes;
    - ○ if no group confirmation, give group O-negative blood.
- **Consider likely source of bleeding** (imaging/surgical input).

10 Post-operative fluids

10.1 FLUID REQUIREMENTS

> **MICRO-facts**
>
> Although gastrointestinal (GI) fluid loss is 200 mL, over 5 litres of fluid is excreted into the GI tract and reabsorbed so anything interfering with this mechanism can lead to extensive fluid loss.

- Normally a balance is maintained between input and output of fluid. This principle is important to remember when prescribing fluids for post-operative patients. The following quantities are the basis for intravenous (IV) fluid therapy.
    - **Input**: maintained by three mechanisms and totals approximately 2500 mL/day:
        - oral fluid intake: 1500 mL;
        - fluid in food: 800 mL;
        - metabolism of food: 200 mL.
    - **Output**: occurs through four main systems:
        - renal tract: 1500 mL;
        - gastrointestinal (GI) tract: 200 mL;
        - insensible losses: 800 mL: (1) respiratory tract; (2) skin.
- Total water content of the body is approximately 42 litres (in a 70 kg man).
- Fluid in the body is not all maintained in one location, it can be divided into three main **compartments**:
    - **Intra-cellular volume**: 28 litres.
    - Extra-cellular volume: 14 litres:
        - **interstitial volume**: 11 litres;
        - **intra-vascular volume**: 3 litres.
- Control of **fluid homeostasis** is via sodium concentration. Increased sodium concentration increases thirst, which in turn increases the production of anti-diuretic hormone (ADH). This leads to increased water reabsorption.

10.2 FLUID COMPARTMENTS

- There are two compartments to consider: intra- and extra-cellular compartments.

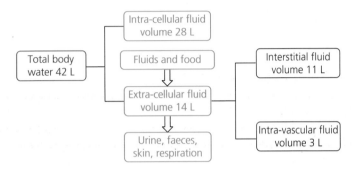

Fig. 10.1 Fluid compartments.

FLUID COMPARTMENT COMPOSITIONS

Extra-cellular fluid (see Table 10.1)

NB value ranges following each electrolyte denote serum concentration.

- Similar in composition to plasma fluid owing to the permeability of the capillary membrane to most dissolved substances except protein.
- The main cation is sodium and the main anion is chloride.
- **Sodium (130–140 mmol/L):**
    - Concentration is maintained by active transport by the sodium: potassium pump (3:2 ratio) on cell membranes.
    - Sodium levels are controlled through the renin–angiotensin system.
    - Sodium requirement is 1 mmol/kg/day.

Table 10.1 Electrolyte concentrations in extra-cellular fluid (ECF) and intra-cellular fluid (ICF)

	ECF (mmol/L)	ICF (mmol/L)
Sodium	140	10
Potassium	4	150
Magnesium	2	123
Chloride	117	10
Calcium	5	0
Bicarbonate	24	8
Phosphate	2	149

On the wards

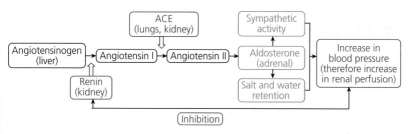

Fig. 10.2 Renin–angiotensin system. ACE, angiotensin-converting enzyme.

Intra-cellular fluid (see Table 10.1)

> **MICRO-print**
> Where there is a low pH, i.e. high levels of hydrogen ions (acidosis), the body will pump hydrogen ions intra-cellularly instead of potassium, creating a hyperkalaemia.

- Cell membranes have more selective membranes so the electrolyte composition is different from that of the extra-cellular fluid (ECF). However, water is able to freely permeate so osmotic pressures are quickly equalized.
- **Potassium (3.5–5.3 mmol/L):**
  - Mainly intra-cellular with 98% of body potassium being contained in the intra-cellular fluid.
  - Factors affecting balance of potassium can be divided into long or short term:
    - **Short:**
      - insulin;
      - pH;
      - β-agonists;
      - bicarbonate concentration.
    - **Long:**
      - the kidney;
      - aldosterone.
  - Potassium is required to maintain the resting membrane potential close to −90 mV; disturbances in extra-cellular potassium can mean the cell is not as responsive to electrical activity. This is a particular problem in conductive pathways in the heart.
  - The Na/K transporter controls the levels of potassium within the intra-cellular fluid as well as sodium.
  - Potassium requirement is also 1 mmol/kg/day.

On the wards

10.3 REPLACEMENT FLUIDS

- Fluids can be divided into colloid or crystalloid.
- Controversy exists concerning the choice of fluid for resuscitation. However, there is limited evidence for benefits of using one over the other.
- Target directed fluid therapy can be used. This involves frequently checking to see whether set targets have been met, e.g. urine output, blood pressure, heart rate.

COLLOID

- These are mainly synthetically produced plasma expanders and albumin solutions.
- Benefits:
  - Large molecules contained within the fluid help it to stay within the vascular system for longer, rather than diffusing into other compartments.
- However, colloids can induce anaphylaxis.

CRYSTALLOID

- These fluids are regularly used in maintenance fluid prescription and can be used for resuscitation (except dextrose).
- They contain electrolytes and water and can be split into isotonic, hypertonic and hypotonic.
- **Hypotonic**: risk of cerebral oedema if used at a high rate/volume:
  - 0.45% saline;
  - 5% dextrose;
  - acts as water because all the dextrose is metabolized.
- **Isotonic**:
  - 0.9% saline;
  - Hartmann's and other 'physiological solutions'.
- **Hypertonic solutions** are used when trying to expand the plasma while not infusing large volumes of fluid:
  - this can be useful when resuscitating those prone to oedema, e.g. burns, extensive bowel surgery;
  - a range of fluids with increased concentrations of sodium.
- The difference between hypotonic and isotonic solutions can be illustrated by comparing distribution between compartments. Sodium is an extra-cellular electrolyte; therefore, sodium-containing fluids are not distributed intra-cellularly, making them effective plasma expanders. Dextrose will not expand the intra-vascular space.
- **Benefits of crystalloids**:
  - cheap in comparison with colloids;
  - less likely to cause a hypersensitivity reaction.

- **Crystalloids** are routinely used for maintenance fluids, the most widely used being:
  - 0.9% saline or 'normal saline';
  - 5% dextrose;
  - compound sodium lactate (Hartmann's solution).
- Their electrolyte compositions are important to remember (Table 10.2).

Table 10.2 Electrolyte compositions of fluids

FLUID	NA$^+$ (mmol/L)	Cl$^-$ (mmol/L)	K$^+$ (mmol/L)	HCO$_3^-$ (mmol/L)	Ca^{2+} (mmol/L)	OSMOLALITY (osm/L)
0.9% saline	154	154	0	0	0	308
5% dextrose	0	0	0	0	0	154
Hartmann's solution	131	112	5	29	4	281

10.4 FLUID PRESCRIBING

RESUSCITATION

- Colloid or crystalloid depending on personal preference.
- **Note: never use 5% dextrose or any solution containing potassium**.

MAINTENANCE

- The requirements are approximately 2500 mL (dependent on a patient's weight, 30 mL/kg/24 h) over 24 hours with approximately 1–2 mmol/kg/day of sodium and 1.0 mmol/kg/day potassium. A common regime is:
  - 1 litre 5% dextrose + 20 mmol of KCl;
  - 1 litre 0.9% saline + 20 mmol of KCl;
  - prescribed over 12 hours.

10.5 FLUID BALANCE ABNORMALITIES

CAUSES OF ABNORMAL FLUID LOSS

- Post-operatively, there are many reasons why patients may lose additional volumes of fluid that require replacement.
- **Additional urinary loss**:
  - Diuretics.
  - Syndrome of inappropriate anti-diuretic hormone secretion (SIADH).
- **Additional GI loss**:
  - Diarrhoea.

On the wards

- Nasogastric tube aspirate.
- GI dysmotility causing fluid sequestration.
- Vomiting.
- **Intra-operative bleeding**: this can be determined by operation notes.
- **Drains at wound sites**.
- **Respiration**.
- **Increased loss in**:
  - Fever/sepsis.
  - Hyperventilation.
  - Burns: owing to loss of skin.
- **Third space loss**:
  - This is an important concept in fluid management.
  - The third space is mainly oedema and transudative loss.
  - Fluid is no longer available to vascular space or metabolic processes. It is an expansion of the ECF, and shares its composition.
  - Fluid sequestered in the third space will start to be reabsorbed after 24–48 hours.
  - Important causes are:
    - oedema at site of surgical injury: this increases with the extent of tissue manipulation the procedure requires;
    - pancreatitis;
    - generalized oedema.
- **Shock (septic/anaphylactic/neurogenic)**:
  - Creates a pseudo-hypovolaemia by extensive vasodilatation.
- **Decreased intake**:
  - Patients are kept nil by mouth prior to surgery and often after surgery.

ASSESSMENT OF FLUID STATUS

- This is structured in the same way as for any other medical consultation with history, examination and investigations. It is important to become skilled at assessing a patient's fluid status as you will be required to do it often.
- **History**:
  - How much?
  - How long?
  - These are the two main questions to discover information about any symptom that will cause increased water loss.
- **Examination**:
  - Thirst.
  - Skin turgor.
  - Dry tongue/mucous membranes.
  - Jugular venous pressure.

- Hypotension/tachycardia.
- Capillary refill time.
- Based on your history and examination you can classify people into mild, moderate or severe (Table 10.3).
- **Investigations**:
  - These can be used to confirm your diagnosis or monitor the success of your fluid prescribing:
    - Urea/creatinine:
      ○ disproportionate rise in urea in dehydration.
    - Haematocrit:
      ○ is a measure of the concentration of red blood cells, therefore increases in dehydration.
    - Urine osmolality.

Table 10.3 Dehydration

DEHYDRATION STATUS	WEIGHT LOSS (% OF TOTAL BODY WEIGHT)	FLUID LOSS IN LITRES (FOR 70 kg MALE)	SIGNS AND SYMPTOMS (CUMULATIVE)
Mild	4	3	Reduced skin turgor, sunken eyes, dry mucous membranes
Moderate	5–8	4–6	Oliguria, hypotension, tachycardia
Severe	8–10	7	Olguria/anuria, decreased cardiovascular system function

REPLACEMENT OF ADDITIONAL FLUID LOSS

- These fluids are in addition to normal maintenance requirement. There are three common causes of fluid depletion:
  - **Blood loss** greater than 15%:
    - replace with blood products.
  - **Blood loss** less than 15%:
    - replace with crystalloid or colloid.
  - **Third space losses after large abdominal surgery**:
    - Hartmann's solution.

On the wards

- Any other additional mechanisms of loss need to be calculated and replaced. Use of central venous pressure and electrolyte results is important as it maintains accuracy.
- After surgery the body is under increased levels of stress, which can lead to increased levels of ADH being produced.
    - This is the **SIADH** (see later under Electrolytes):
        - This can be confusing as urine output is low or absent but the patient is well hydrated and therefore at risk of fluid overload.
        - Normally this can be treated with fluid restriction in a medical patient.
        - However, this is not possible post-operatively; 5% dextrose should be avoided as it will worsen hyponatraemia.

FLUID CHALLENGE

- Fluid challenges can be used to differentiate types of shock.
- A response to the fluid challenge (slow increase in blood pressure and decrease in heart rate) indicates the patient is hypovolaemic. No response after 2 litres of fluid shows that the patient's primary problem is unlikely to be hypovolaemia and may indicate septic shock or active bleeding.

MICRO-techniques
FLUID CHALLENGE
1. Gain intravenous access. A large-bore cannula (16G or larger) should be used.
2. Attach a three-way tap to the cannula.
3. To one port attach a bag of 0.9% saline and to the other, attach a 50 mL syringe.
4. Fill the syringe with 50 mL of saline and deliver this to the patient as rapidly as possible. Repeat this until 250 mL has been given.
5. Assess the patient's fluid status (respiratory rate, chest auscultation, heart rate, blood pressure).
6. Repeat up to 2 litres of fluid if the chest remains clear and there are no signs of fluid overload.

10.6 ELECTROLYTES

SODIUM

Hyponatraemia (serum sodium <130 mmol/L)

- Hyponatraemia is a common finding among inpatients.
- **Signs and symptoms** (usually when Na^+ below 115 mmol/L) include:
    - nausea and vomiting;
    - visual disturbances;

- confusion, decreased consciousness, coma;
- seizures, muscle cramps, myoclonus.

- Hyponatraemia may occur in either hypo-/hyper- or euvolaemic states. Accurate establishment of the cause is essential as treatment involves either water restriction or addition of saline.
- Hyponatraemia may occur via depletion or dilution:
  - **Depletion** occurs when the body is losing water but losing greater amounts of sodium:
    - Treatment is via administration of saline as these patients are **hypovolaemic**.
    - Depletion can occur via renal loss or loss from elsewhere:
      - ○ **Renal** causes will be distinguished by high urinary sodium. Common causes include: diuretics; hypoadrenalism (Addison's disease); renal tubular acidosis; salt-losing nephropathies.
      - ○ **Extra-renal** causes can be distinguished by low urinary sodium. Common causes include: diarrhoea; vomiting; third-space losses.
  - **Dilution** occurs when the body is retaining fluid, giving a low serum sodium without a reduction in total body sodium:
    - Treatment is via **fluid restriction**.
    - This can occur when **hypervolaemic** or when **euvolaemic**:
      - ○ **Hypervolaemic** situations can be distinguished by the presence of oedema. Common causes include: congestive cardiac failure; cirrhosis; nephrotic syndrome; overdose of IV fluid, in particular 5% dextrose.
    - **Euvolaemic** situations have a low plasma osmolality, caused by slight increase in ECF volume and normal sodium. Common causes include: SIADH (urine osmolality > 500 mmol/L); inappropriate fluids (urine osmolality < 500 mmol/L); renal failure (urine osmolality < 500 mmol/L); hypothyroidism (urine osmolality < 500 mmol/L).

MICRO-print
The syndrome of inappropriate anti-diuretic hormone secretion (SIADH) is an inability to suppress the levels of ADH secreted. Higher levels of ADH increase the concentration of functioning aquaporins in the collecting ducts. This leads to retention of water and hyponatraemia. Major surgery is one of the causes of SIADH, as is small cell lung cancer, drugs, central nervous system disturbances and human immunodeficiency virus. Treatment involves water restriction and occasionally a tetracycline derivative – demeclocycline.

On the wards

Hypernatraemia (serum sodium >150 mmol/L)

- The increase in plasma sodium levels means there is intra-cellular dehydration because the ECF is hyperosmolar. This accounts for many signs and symptoms.
- **Signs and symptoms** include (severity depends on speed of onset):
  - Pyrexia.
  - Nausea and vomiting.
  - Convulsions and coma.
  - Any neurological disturbance.
- Hypernatraemia may occur with a reduction in intake of fluid, excessive loss or excessive gain of sodium:
  - **Lack of fluid intake**.
  - **Excessive fluid loss**, can be due to a pre-renal or renal cause:
    - **Pre-renal**:
      - ○ fever;
      - ○ hyperventilation;
      - ○ vomiting;
      - ○ diarrhoea.
    - **Renal causes**:
      - ○ **Osmotic diuresis**: this is caused by having another solute, resulting in hyperosmolality, e.g. diabetic ketoacidosis (DKA); hyperosmolar non-ketotic coma; mannitol administration.
      - ○ **Diabetes insipidus**: abnormal production of or response to ADH, e.g. central; nephrogenic.
  - **Excessive salt intake**:
    - Iatrogenic, excessive saline administration.
    - Excessive steroids.
    - Iatrogenic.
    - Cushing's syndrome.
- **Investigation** of hypernatraemia is a combination of four variables:
  - Volume status.
  - Urine osmolality.
  - Plasma osmolality.
  - Urine output.
- If the patient is euvolaemic or hypervolaemic then the most likely cause is excessive salt intake.
- If the patient is hypovolaemic then they are losing water in excess of salt, or have no water intake.
- **Treatment of hypernatraemia** is dependent on the volume status but is based on IV fluid therapy.
  - Patients who are not volume deplete can have their deficit in water replaced by 5% dextrose.

- Patients who are volume deplete can be rehydrated with normal saline, which will be hypotonic for them as they are running in a hypertonic state.

> **MICRO-facts**
>
> Both hypo- and hypernatraemia should be considered in view of fluid status, for example
> - hypovolaemic
> - euvolaemic
> - hyperkalaemic

POTASSIUM

Hypokalaemia (serum potassium 3.5 mmol/L)

- The body cannot alter the loss of potassium through the kidney as efficiently as sodium, so hypokalaemia can occur rapidly.
- **Signs and symptoms**:
  - anorexia and nausea;
  - muscle weakness;
  - paralytic ileus.
- **ECG signs**:
  - ST depression;
  - reduced T wave height;
  - a U wave;
  - widened QRS.

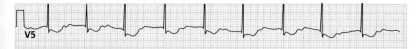

Fig. 10.3 Hypokalaemia ECG.

- Causes of hypokalaemia can be divided into increased loss through the kidneys or redistribution of body potassium into cells. Reduced intake is very rare.
- **Increased loss**:
  - diarrhoea, nausea, vomiting;
  - diuretics;
  - hyperaldosteronism;
  - Conn's syndrome, Cushing's syndrome;
  - renal artery stenosis;
  - renal tubular acidosis;
  - renal failure.

On the wards

- **Redistribution**:
    - insulin administration;
    - β_2 agonists (e.g. salbutamol).
- **Investigation**:
    - If the cause is not iatrogenic, then a measurement of urinary potassium will be diagnostically useful.
    - If >40 mmol/L then the loss is renal and all the renal causes can be investigated.
    - If <40 mmol/L then the loss is probably occurring from the GI tract.

MICRO-facts

It is essential to put a limit on any prescription of oral potassium. If not, you may well end up treating hyperkalaemia as a result.

- **Treatment**:
    - Replacement of potassium and treatment of the underlying cause. However, the route varies on the profundity of the deficit:
        - **Less than 2.5 mmol/L**: IV KCl in 1 litre of fluid at a rate not exceeding 20 mmol/h and concentration not exceeding 40 mmol/L.
        - **Greater than 2.5 mmol/L**: oral supplements will be adequate. The exceptions are if the patient is at risk of arrythmias (e.g. after myocardial infarction or previous history) or if the patient is still vomiting or not taking oral medications.

Hyperkalaemia (serum potassium >5.5 mmol/L)

MICRO-facts

ECG changes as a result of hyperkalaemia indicate a medical emergency and treatment should be instigated without waiting for a potassium level.

- **Signs and symptoms**:
    - muscle weakness.
- **ECG changes**:
    - T wave peaking;
    - broad QRS;
    - prolonged PR;
    - loss of P waves;
    - sine wave appearance.

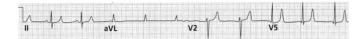

Fig. 10.4 Hyperkalaemia ECG.

- Causes of **hyperkalaemia** can be divided into impaired excretion, redistribution and excessive intake:
  - **Impaired excretion**:
    - renal failure;
    - Addison's disease;
    - potassium-sparing diuretics.

MICRO-facts

Potassium levels can be falsely elevated by: tourniquet use, haemolysis in sampling, exercise. If a level is unexpectedly high then it is important to repeat the test.

  - **Redistribution**:
    - burns, trauma;
    - tumour necrosis;
    - haemolysis;
    - GI bleed.
  - **Excessive intake**:
    - inappropriate prescription of potassium;
    - blood transfusions.
- **Investigations**:
  - The most important investigation is an **ECG** to check for effect on the myocardium.
  - A venous blood sample can also be analysed on a blood gas analyser quickly.
- **Treatment** (in the absence of ECG changes) varies on the level of hyperkalaemia and local protocol:
  - **Less than ~6.0 mmol/L**: potassium restriction.
  - **Greater than ~6.5 mmol/L**:
    - 10 mL of calcium gluconate 10% IV over 2 minutes stabilizes the myocardium;
    - administration of insulin (10 units short-acting) to encourage cellular uptake, and glucose (50 mL of 50%) to prevent hypoglycaemia;
    - salbutamol nebulisers.
  - If hyperkalaemia continues dialysis may be required.

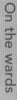

On the wards

CALCIUM (2.12–2.65 mmol/L)

> **MICRO-print**
> Corrected calcium = (0.8 × (normal albumin − patient's albumin)) + serum Ca

- **Daily requirement**: 0.05–0.1 mmol/kg/day.
- Although the majority (99%) of calcium is present in the bones and teeth, when in the blood it is ionized, non-ionized or bound to plasma proteins.
- Ionized calcium is the active form; therefore, it is important to know that fraction of the serum calcium, usually called adjusted calcium.
- Calcium is involved in **muscle contraction**, as well as other body systems.
- Calcium levels are controlled by **parathyroid hormone**, **vitamin D**, **calcitonin** and **thyroxine**.
- It is excreted through the kidney and GI tract.

Hypercalcaemia (serum calcium > 2.5 mmol/L)

- Can present with changes in mental state, formation of kidney stones, diarrhoea and conduction disorders.
- **ECG changes** include shortening of the QT or PR interval and widening of the QRS.
- Causes include:
    - primary and tertiary hyperparathyroidism;
    - hyperthyroidism;
    - immobility;
    - malignancy;
    - renal failure.
- **Treatment** involves rehydration with normal saline; IV bisphosphonates can also be used or dialysis in severe cases.

> **MICRO-facts**
> The adage: **groans**, **stones**, **bones** and **psychiatric moans** can be useful in remembering the classical signs of hypercalcaemia.

Hypocalcaemia (serum calcium < 2 mmol/L)

- Can also present with changes to mental state, as with hypercalcaemia, as well as tetany, spasm and Chvostek's and Trousseau's signs.
- **ECG changes** include lengthening of the QT interval, developing into heart block.

On the wards

MICRO-facts

- **Chvostek's sign**: tapping over the facial nerve causes facial spasm.
- **Trousseau's sign**: inflating a blood pressure cuff to above the level of the systolic blood pressure for 3 minutes causes muscle spasms in the hand and forearm.

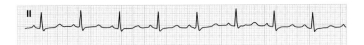

Fig. 10.5 Hypocalcaemia ECG.

- **Causes** include:
  - Secondary hyperparathyroidism.
  - Hypoalbuminaemia:
    - poor protein intake;
    - sepsis;
    - burns;
    - extensive transfusion.
- **Treatment** involves replacement of calcium with either calcium gluconate or calcium carbonate.

MICRO-print

The mechanism of calcium transport in the serum can be illustrated by an asthma or panic attack. With increased respiration, patients blow off their carbon dioxide which alters their pH and makes them alkalotic. This means there is less ionization of calcium and the symptoms of hypocalcaemia present.

MAGNESIUM (serum magnesium 0.75–1.00 mmol/L)

- Requirement 0.08–0.2 mmol/kg/day.
- The distribution of magnesium in the body is: 65% in bones and 25% in cells.
- Magnesium is involved in adenosine triphosphate (ATP) production as well as nucleic acid formation.

Hypomagnesaemia (serum magnesium <0.70 mmol/L)

> **MICRO-facts**
>
> If you are treating low potassium or calcium and the levels are not rising, it is important to check the level of magnesium as low potassium or calcium levels will not rise in the presence of low levels of magnesium.

- Can present with symptoms similar to hypocalcaemia, i.e. weakness, anorexia and Chvostek's and Trousseau's signs.
- It often also presents with hypocalcaemia, and hypokalaemia.
- **Causes** include:
    - diarrhoea;
    - malabsorption;
    - diuretics;
    - alcohol excess;
    - post-acute tubular necrosis;
    - post-renal transplantation;
    - post-diuresis after obstruction.
- **ECG changes** can include broad QRS and peaked T waves.
- **Treatment** revolves around magnesium replacement via oral or IV routes.

Hypermagnesaemia (serum magnesium <1.05 mmol/L)

> **MICRO-facts**
>
> Large doses of magnesium are often administered as treatment for smooth muscle relaxation effects; for example, asthma, depression of the central nervous system, e.g. in pre-eclampsia, or cardiac stabilization, e.g. arrhythmias. These treatments have been linked with hypermagnesaemia in only isolated cases.

- This is rare, because magnesium is poorly absorbed through the small bowel. However, magnesium is mainly excreted through the renal system; therefore, patients with kidney failure are at risk of retaining magnesium.
- **Signs and symptoms**:
    - include hyporeflexia, somnolence, muscle paralysis, bradycardia and hypotension.
- **Causes**:
    - magnesium enemas;
    - laxative abuse.

- **ECG changes** include elongation of PR, broadening of the QRS and elongation of the QT.
- **Treatment** is mainly through dialysis; however, in an emergency, IV calcium can be administered. Anticipation of problems in patients with renal failure can avoid hypermagnesaemia becoming a problem.

PHOSPHATE (0.8–1.5 mmol/L)

- Requirement 0.2–0.5 mmol/kg per day.
- Phosphate is the key intra-cellular anion, and is involved in the production of ATP and nucleic acids.
- Phosphate absorption from the gut is increased by the action of parathyroid hormone (PTH) and vitamin D. Absorption from the gut is unregulated unless it is bound by cations, e.g. magnesium or calcium.
- Phosphate is mainly excreted renally, which can increase excretion to cope with all but the largest of phosphate loads.

Hyperphosphataemia (serum phosphate > 1.5 mmol/L)

- The main consequence of high levels of phosphate is to cause hypocalcaemia via suppression of calcitriol, so the **signs and symptoms** are similar to those of hypocalcaemia.
- **Causes** include:
  - **Acute phosphate load**:
    - Rhabdomyolysis.
    - Tumour lysis.
    - Ketoacidosis.
  - **Renal failure**:
    - Inability to excrete phosphate.
  - **Hypoparathyroidism**:
    - PTH causes reabsorption of phosphate in the distal tubule.
- **ECG changes**:
  - Similar to hypercalcaemia.
- **Treatment**:
  - Dependent on whether the high phosphate is acute or chronic:
    - **Acute**: saline infusion can increase excretion if renal function is normal. If not then dialysis can help.
    - **Chronic**: phosphate binders to decrease absorption in the gut and a low-phosphate diet.

Hypophosphataemia (serum phosphate < 0.8 mmol/L)

- Disorders causing low phosphate:
  - Osteomalacia, rickets, rhabdomyolysis, encephalopathy, congestive heart failure, proximal myopathy and haemolysis.
- **Urinary phosphate** can be a good biomarker to delineate between causes if the reason is not clear from the history.

On the wards

- **Signs and symptoms**:
  - Irritability.
  - Shortness of breath.
  - Seizures.
  - Delirium and coma.
- **Causes**:
  - **Redistribution**:
    - refeeding syndrome: caused by insulin release;
    - insulin administration in DKA;
    - respiratory alkalosis.
  - **Decreased absorption**:
    - diarrhoea;
    - starvation;
    - alcoholism;
    - magnesium salt ingestion.
  - **Increased urinary loss**:
    - hyperparathyroidism.
- **Treatment**:
  - Replacement of phosphate either orally or intravenously.
  - If vitamin D deficiency is thought to be the cause then supplements can help.

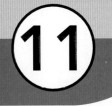

Recognizing and managing ill patients

11.1 INTRODUCTION

A major part of a junior doctor's work involves being called to see acutely unwell patients on the wards. This can initially be a daunting task. It should be remembered that most critical illnesses do not occur instantly; the junior doctor has time to act before calling for help (Table 11.1).

The following few pages give a brief outline of the process to follow in an acute situation. Throughout the country 'early warning scoring' systems have been developed. These systems attribute scores to a set of observations dependent on their extent of deviation from the norm.

On the wards

Table 11.1 ABCDE assessment

AIRWAY	BREATHING	CIRCULATION	DISABILITY	EXPOSURE
• **Look:** • Fogging of mask • Inside the mouth • Symmetrical movement of the chest with respiration • Abdominal breathing ("seesaw" breathing) • **Listen:** • Talk to the patient • Gurgling/Stridor/Wheeze • Silence • **Feel:** • Feel for breath on the palm/cheek • **Action:** • Suction • Airway manoeuvres: head tilt-chin lift/raw thrust • Airway adjuncts: Guedel, nasopharyngeal tube, laryngeal mask, endotracheal tube (intubation)	• **Look:** • Observations: RR, saturations • Thorax movement: symmetrical/asymmetrical • Colour: evidence of cyanosis • Use of accessory muscles of respiration: subcostal and intercostal recession • Lip pursing • Nasal flaring • Patient's position: sat up, leaning forwards, lying • **Listen:** • Percuss the chest: resonant, dull • Auscultate the chest: front and back – vesicular breath sounds, wheeze, crepitations, silence • **Feel:** • Tracheal deviation • Chest expansion	• **Look:** • HR, BP • Urine output – marker of renal perfusion. Should be at least 0.5 mL/kg/h • Conscious level – marker of cerebral perfusion • Colour • Jugular venous pressure • **Listen:** • Heart sounds • **Feel:** • Temperature of peripheries • Pulse: rhythm, character and rate • Capillary refill time • Skin turgor • Apex beat • Calf swelling or tenderness • Peripheral oedema	• **Pupils:** size and light reflexes • **Glasgow coma scale score/ AVPU** • **Brief neurology examination** • **BM** (don't ever forget glucose) • **Action:** • O_2 • If hypoglycaemic, administer glucose • Airway protection of P or U on the AVPU scale • Exclude profound hypotension, hypercapnia, medication • Further investigation, i.e. CT head	• **Take a brief history:** • Timing and onset and nature of symptoms • Pain history • **Review observation chart** once more • **Review all other charts,** i.e. stool charts, fluid balance charts • **Review drug chart** • **Read patient notes** – establish: • Reason for current admission • Current inpatient problems and current treatment and investigation plan • Background: PMH, previous surgery • Baseline function, i.e. where live when not in hospital, level of care need, dependants

Get help: anaesthetics/ cardiac arrest team	• **Action:**	• **Action:**	• **Examine the following systems** depending on the history taken:
	• 15 litres of oxygen via a non-rebreathe mask (reservoir mask)	• IV access: 2 × large-bore cannulas in each antecubital fossa	• GI examination
	• Bag and mask: supplement a low respiratory rate or maintain breaths in a patient making no respiratory effort	• Bloods: should be taken when the cannula is inserted. FBC, U&Es, LFTs, lactate, cross-match match, blood cultures	• Inspect the patient for rashes/other skin changes
	• Call for help: cardiac arrest team	• Fluid challenge	• Brief musculoskeletal examination if indicated
		• Catheterize: allows for accurate monitoring of urine output	• Examine the head for trauma
		• Call for help. If no improvement after 3 litres of fluid is given, patient must be considered for escalation of care to HDU/ITU where inotropic support of blood pressure can be delivered	• Inspect all lines going into patient
			• Note output from all drains/stomas: content and amount

AVPU, Alert, Voice, Pain, Unresponsive score; BM, blood sugar level; FBC, full blood count; GI, gastrointestinal; HDU, high dependency unit; ITU, intensive therapy unit; LFT, liver function tests; PMH, previous medical history; U&Es, urea and electrolytes.

(a)

	3	**2**	**1**	**0**	**1**	**2**	**3**
Conscious level			New confusion or agitation	Awake	Responds to voice		Responds to pain or unconscious
Respiratory rate	Less than 8	8		9–18	19–24	25–29	30 or more
Heart rate	40 or less	41–49		50–100	101–115	116–129	130 or more
Systolic BP	70 or less	71–80	81–100	101–199		200 or more	
Temperature		35°c or less	35.1°c–35.9°c	36°c–37.9°c	38°c–38.9°c	39°c or above	
SpO$_2$ – on O$_2$ therapy	85% or less	86–89%					
Urine output	Any patient scoring 3 or above may require urine output monitoring. If catheterized, consider hourly catchments. If not catheterized, consider whether a urinary catheter is necessary.						

(b)

Guidelines

If a patient scores 3 on a combination of parameters the nurse in charge must be informed. He/she will decide on appropriate action and whether a referral is necessary

A patient who scores 3 on any single parameter or 4 on a combination of parameters should be referred to medical team/outreach/night matrons. The nurse in charge must also be made aware

If a patient's condition is of concern to you and they are not triggering an EWS score, do not hesitate to contact outreach for advice or support

Fig. 11.1 Example of early warning scoring (EWS) system and guidelines. BP, blood pressure.

MICRO-facts

EWS are population specific, e.g. EWS designed for adults will be completely different to an obstetric EWS.

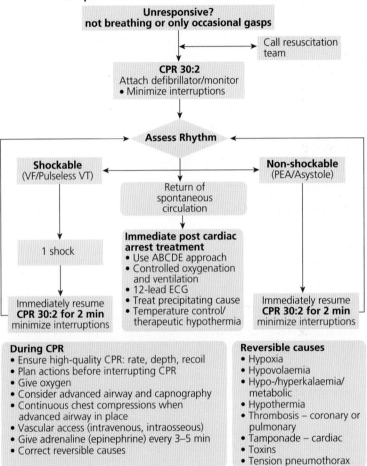

**Adult ALS (Advanced Life Support) cardiac arrest algorithm
European Resuscitation Council Guidelines 2010**

**Unresponsive?
not breathing or only occasional gasps**

Call resuscitation team

CPR 30:2
Attach defibrillator/monitor
• Minimize interruptions

Assess Rhythm

Shockable
(VF/Pulseless VT)

Non-shockable
(PEA/Asystole)

Return of spontaneous circulation

1 shock

Immediate post cardiac arrest treatment
• Use ABCDE approach
• Controlled oxygenation and ventilation
• 12-lead ECG
• Treat precipitating cause
• Temperature control/ therapeutic hypothermia

Immediately resume
CPR 30:2 for 2 min
minimize interruptions

Immediately resume
CPR 30:2 for 2 min
minimize interruptions

During CPR
• Ensure high-quality CPR: rate, depth, recoil
• Plan actions before interrupting CPR
• Give oxygen
• Consider advanced airway and capnography
• Continuous chest compressions when advanced airway in place
• Vascular access (intravenous, intraosseous)
• Give adrenaline (epinephrine) every 3–5 min
• Correct reversible causes

Reversible causes
• Hypoxia
• Hypovolaemia
• Hypo-/hyperkalaemia/ metabolic
• Hypothermia
• Thrombosis – coronary or pulmonary
• Tamponade – cardiac
• Toxins
• Tension pneumothorax

Fig. 11.2 Resuscitation guidelines. Reproduced from Resuscitation Council UK (2010) Adult Advanced Life Support Algorithm.

On the wards

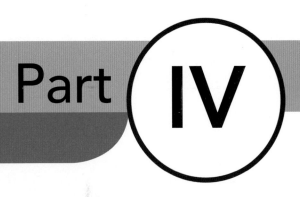

Part IV

Intensive therapy unit/ critical care

VI

Intensive therapy units/critical care

Structure of an intensive therapy unit

12.1 INTRODUCTION

- Intensive therapy is the highest level of care that a hospital can provide (Table 12.1). It is run by anaesthetists or intensivists and has a very small number of beds (approximately 1–2% of the total beds in the hospital).
- The requirement for intensive therapy is 1:1 nursing care. This is defined as level 3 care, with level 2 being a high dependency unit, level 1 being a specialist ward (e.g. coronary care unit) and level 0 being normal wards.
- With the small number of beds available, the resource of intensive therapy is directed towards people who have a potentially recoverable condition and who would benefit the most from high-level care.

Table 12.1 Levels of care in a hospital

LEVEL OF CARE	CRITERIA
Level 0	Requires hospitalization Observations required no more than 4 hourly
Level 1	Recent discharge from a higher level Staff with extra expertise Additional monitoring required
Level 2	Single organ support Pre-operative optimization Post-operative monitoring More frequent observations Step down from a higher level
Level 3	Advanced respiratory support Advanced cardiovascular support Two organ systems supported

12.2 ADMISSION

- The categories of people who require intensive therapy unit (ITU) level support have:
  - respiratory failure;
  - failure of two or more organ systems.
- The main **organ systems** that can be supported in ITU are:
  - **respiratory**;
  - **cardiovascular**;
  - **renal**;
  - **neurological**.
- Admission to ITU is usually a consultant-to-consultant referral. The suitability of applying the resources of ITU to a patient must be assessed by a clinician with the knowledge and experience to decide whether the patient would benefit.
- Chronic ill health cannot be improved by ITU. However, if people with co-morbidities have become accustomed to a quality of life others would find unacceptable, then they remain candidates for assessment.
- Patients with sepsis are a good example of people who benefit from the intensive therapy and organ support that can be offered. Sepsis will be used as an example when discussing organ support.
- If it is anticipated that a patient will require ITU intervention, then there is often an anaesthetic registrar who covers the wards as outreach and will assess the suitability of the patient for ITU and anticipated further management.

MICRO-print

Hepatic dysfunction can be supported by management of coagulopathy. Dermatological dysfunction can also be managed after severe burns, with asepsis and preventing excess fluid loss.

12.3 STAFF

CONSULTANT

- There will always be a consultant intensivist on call for ITU.
- The consultant's level of experience will enable him or her to make decisions about outcome and the possible success of treatment and to advise on admission to the unit.

MEDICAL STAFF ON THE UNIT

- Various grades of doctor from second year junior to registrar have roles as communicators and clinicians.

- As a **communicator** they act as an information conduit. Patients may have many specialists providing input and it is important to have personnel to assimilate the information, present it to the consultant at ward round and keep specialist teams informed of the current management plan.
- As a **clinician**, each patient needs:
    - assessment when they enter ITU;
    - daily review;
    - review when physiological parameters change.

ITU NURSING STAFF

- Nurses in ITU have a vast amount of experience and training and are mainly responsible for the care of the patient. There is one nurse for each patient, and an additional nurse to carry out administrative duties.
- Nurses are able to:
    - manage fluid replacement;
    - wean off ventilation;
    - provide analgesia.
- In addition to specialist care, general care includes:
    - washing;
    - turning;
    - frequent and accurate charting of patient observations including fluid balance.

MICROBIOLOGIST

- Intensive monitoring of patients from a microbiology perspective is essential.
- The intensive monitoring that patients require means there are many indwelling lines, cannulas and catheters, which are areas for growth of multiresistant organisms.
- Microbiologists make daily ward rounds of ITU to review the latest swabs, cultures and other samples taken from patients.
- To limit the development of resistant species certain antibiotics require a code obtained from microbiology. These are mainly broad-spectrum, non-specific antibacterial agents that are avoided if more specific antibiotics can be used, which is guided by culture and sensitivities.

PHYSIOTHERAPY

Physiotherapists have a number of techniques that are commonly used among ITU patients:
- Positioning:
    - the avoidance of pressure sores due to immobility.

Intensive therapy unit/critical care

- Further mobilization:
  - can help redistribute fluid, and improve alveolar ventilation; limb exercises can also help to retain range of motion in joints.
- Chest physiotherapy:
  - percussion and vibration can help to move secretions in the patient's chest;
  - suction also helps with upper airways secretion.
- Manual hyperinflation (taking the patient off the ventilator and providing a large tidal volume):
  - improves alveolar recruitment.

DIETICIAN

- While in ITU patients are often unable to take food because of decreased consciousness or respiratory support systems.
- The stress response from surgery, sepsis or trauma activates inflammatory processes and leads to a catabolic, hyperglycaemic state with increased lipolysis.
- Early enteral feeding can be helpful in improving the outcome of patients. There are few contraindications to this, the most notable being gastrointestinal obstruction or ileus.

PHARMACIST

- The number and variety of medications used by an intensive therapy unit often requires the input of a pharmacist.
- The pharmacist can be involved in drug dosing, rationalization of drug therapy, reduction in prescribing errors, efficacy of therapies and financial savings.

Intensive therapy unit/critical care

13

Principles of critical care

13.1 ORGAN SUPPORT

RESPIRATORY

- People who receive assistance with their ventilation are:
  - Hypoxic.
  - Hypercapnic.
  - Anticipated to become exhausted.
- For **hypoxic** patients a stepwise increase in therapy would be:
  - Oxygen via a face mask (40%, 50%, 60%).
  - Continual positive airway pressure ventilation.
  - Mechanical ventilation.
- Patients who are **hypercapnic** also require respiratory support. CO_2 is cleared only if there is increased alveolar ventilation, so non-invasive ventilation is first-line therapy if the patient is becoming acidotic with oxygen therapy.
  - These can be negative or positive pressure forms of ventilation:
    - **Non-invasive positive pressure ventilation (NIPPV)**:
      - delivers synchronized positive pressure breaths via a nasal or mouth mask;
      - BiPAP is a form of NIPPV that provides two levels of positive pressure with a lower one at expiration.
    - **Negative pressure ventilation**:
      - cycles between a negative pressure and atmospheric pressure.
- If carbon dioxide continues to rise by 7 kPa or 2 kPa above the patient's normal level then mechanical ventilation is often required.

MICRO-facts

Continuous positive airway pressure (CPAP) is only appropriate if the patient is making a respiratory effort, is alert, does not have a basal skull injury and is not at risk of aspiration. Many patients find CPAP uncomfortable and claustrophobic, which will require escalation of treatment.

CARDIOVASCULAR

- Support for the cardiovascular system should be considered once there is adequate respiratory support.
- A septic patient will often require cardiovascular support owing to peripheral vasodilatation and decrease in cardiac contractility.
- There are five mechanisms that can be adjusted when optimizing cardiovascular support:
    - pre-load;
    - contractility;
    - heart rate;
    - heart rhythm;
    - afterload.
- The cardiovascular system can be monitored via:
    - ECG;
    - arterial blood pressure;
    - pulmonary artery pressure;
    - pulmonary capillary wedge pressure;
    - urine output;
    - central venous pressure.

Pre-load

- Pre-load can be adjusted via intravenous fluid therapy if deplete, or diuretics if overloaded.
- Vasodilators are also important (Table 13.1) (see later under Afterload).

Contractility

- Contractility can be affected by:
    - Drugs:
        - increasing cyclic adenosine monophosphate (cAMP) availability;
        - decreasing breakdown of cAMP, phosphodiesterase inhibitors;
        - increasing calcium availability, e.g. glucagon, digoxin;
        - increasing the reaction to calcium, e.g. levosimendan.
    - Oxygen.
    - Fluids.
- Inotropes or catecholamines act by affecting cAMP, which affects adrenoreceptors; there are four main types of receptor that are located in different areas of the body (Table 13.2).
- Four of the main catecholamines are listed in Table 13.3.
- These drugs can be used be used in isolation or combination. For example, in septic shock the myocardium is depressed so dobutamine is good at increasing cardiac output; however, there is also vasodilatation, which can be decreased by noradrenaline.

Table 13.1 Drugs effecting afterload or pre-load

CLASS OF DRUG	EXAMPLES	MODE OF ACTION	PRE-LOAD	AFTER-LOAD	COMMENTS
Nitrates	GTN ISMN	Decrease intra-cellular calcium	✓		Tolerance develops after 24 hours; nitrates are absorbed by plastic
Potassium channel agonists	Hydralazine Minoxidil Nicorandil	Activate the ATP K^+ channel, causing muscular relaxation		✓	Nicorandil works in this fashion but also stimulates nitrate release, which means that it affects both pre-load and afterload
Calcium channel blocker	Nifedipine Felodipine Amlodipine	Reduce calcium intake through long-acting voltage-gated channels		✓	These are mainly the second- and third-generation calcium channel blockers
AT_1 blockers	Losartan Candesartan Irbesartan	Block AT_1, blocking the action of angiotensin II		✓	They have a long half-life as they are highly protein bound. May also cause hyperkalaemia when administered with K^+-sparing diuretics
ACE inhibitors	Ramipril Enalapril Lisinopril	Inhibit the formation of angiotensin II by ACE, which is a vasoconstrictor	✓	✓	ACE inhibitors are also involved in bradykinin production, which can cause a dry cough

Intensive therapy unit/critical care

Table 13.1 (*Continued*)

CLASS OF DRUG	EXAMPLES	MODE OF ACTION	PRE-LOAD	AFTER-LOAD	COMMENTS
α-blockers	Adrenaline Nor-adrenaline	Stimulate α-receptors in smooth muscle	✓	✓	

ACE, angiotensin-converting enzyme; AT_1, angiotensin II receptor type 1; GTN, glyceryl trinitrate; ISMN, isosorbide mononitrate.

Table 13.2 Catecholamine receptors

RECEPTORS	LOCATION	ACTION
α	Peripheral, renal, cardiac	Vasoconstriction
β_1	Cardiac	Increase contraction and cardiac output
β_2	Peripheral and renal	Vasodilation
Dopamine receptors	Renal, gastrointestinal, cardiac	With increasing doses: vasodilation, myocardial contraction, vasoconstriction

Table 13.3 Effects of catecholamines on adrenergic receptors

DRUG	α	β_1	β_2	EFFECT	WHEN USED
Dobutamine	0	3	2	↑CO and ↓afterload	Ischaemic heart disease
Adrenaline	1–3	3	2	↑CO and ↓SVR	Cardiac arrest, anaphylaxis
Noradrenaline	3	1	0	Vasoconstriction	Vasodilatation-induced hypotension

0, no effect; 1, minimal effect; 2, moderate effect; 3, large effect.

Heart rate

- Heart rate can be increased or decreased to optimize output.
- Drugs which increase heart rate (positive chronotropes):
    - Parasympathetic antagonists, e.g. atropine.
    - Sympathetic agonists that affect β_1, e.g. dobutamine, adrenaline.
    - Dihydropyridine calcium channel blockers, e.g. amlodipine, nifedipine; cause vasodilatation, hypotension and a reflex tachycardia.

- Drugs which will decrease heart rate (negative inotropes):
  - Sympathetic antagonists:
    - β-blockers, e.g. atenolol, bisoprolol.
  - Non-dihydropyridine calcium channel blockers, e.g. diltiazem, verapamil.
    - negative inotropic effects.

MICRO-facts

Administration of a calcium channel blocker such as verapamil to a supraventricular tachycardia caused by Wolff–Parkinson–White (WPW) syndrome can lead to ventricular tachycardia. This is because blockade at the atrioventricular node allows all the action potentials to travel along the aberrant pathway with no rate limit. For this reason calcium channel blockers are not used in WPW.

Heart rhythm

- The rhythm should ideally be optimized to achieve maximal cardiac output.
- Patients in the intensive therapy unit (ITU) are at risk of arrhythmias because of:
  - electrolyte imbalance;
  - hypoxia/hypercapnia;
  - hypotension;
  - iatrogenic, e.g. catecholamine administration, line insertion.
- Anti-arrythmics are organized into classes 1–4 (Table 13.4).
- There are two commonly used anti-arrhythmic drugs that are not in the classification.
- **Adenosine** acts by decreasing cAMP and K^+ channel blocking. It is used for converting supraventricular tachycardias to sinus rhythm.
- **Digoxin** is an organically derived compound. The mechanism of action is unclear; however, it does inhibit the Na/K channel. It can be used for controlling atrial fibrillation when there is insufficient blood pressure for a β-blocker, as it does not decrease blood pressure.

MICRO-facts

Digoxin has a narrow therapeutic range. Toxicity can be shown on the ECG by a downward sloping ST segment (reverse tick) and T wave inversion. This can be confused with ischaemia. To check digoxin levels, serum has to be taken at 6–8 hours after the dose.

Intensive therapy unit/critical care

Table 13.4 Anti-arrhythmic drugs

DRUG CLASS	EXAMPLES	MECHANISM OF ACTION	ARRHYTHMIAS
Class 1a	Quinidine Disopyramide	Na^+ channel blocker (moderate)	WPW syndrome Prevention of SVT, VF, VT
Class 1b	Lignocaine Mexiletine	Na^+ channel blocker (mild)	Prevention of VF, VT (in ischaemia)
Class 1c	Flecainide	Na^+ channel blocker (severe)	Conversion of SVT, AF, VF, VT
Class 2	Atenolol Bisoprolol Propranolol	β-blockade	Rate control of AF Prevention of SVT, VF, VT
Class 3	Amiodarone Sotalol	K^+ channel blockers	Prevention of SVT, VF, VT
Class 4	Diltiazem Verapamil	Calcium channel blockers	Rate control of AF

AF, atrial fibrillation; SVT, supraventricular tachycardia; VF, ventricular fibrillation; VT, ventricular tachycardia; WPW, Wolff–Parkinson–White.

Afterload

- Afterload is determined by SVR.
- The main conditions which require modification of afterload are:
  - left ventricular failure;
  - hypertension;
  - ischaemic heart disease.
- Systemic vascular resistance can be decreased by vasodilators that affect either arteries or veins, or both (Table 13.1).

RENAL

- Renal injury is common in patients in ITU owing to their mechanisms of presentation. Kidneys require a high level of oxygenation and perfusion to function. Any dysfunction of respiratory or cardiovascular systems can lead to acute kidney injury/failure.
- A septic patient will become hypotensive as a result of vasodilatation, which will cause a period of kidney hypoperfusion until fluid resuscitation occurs. The hypoperfusion will lead to hypoxia and acute tubular necrosis.
- Prior to renal replacement therapy there are other measures that can be used to try and **maintain renal function**; they include:

- treating hypovolaemia, maintaining mean arterial pressure (MAP), cardiac output and oxygen saturation;
- stopping any nephrotoxic drugs if possible;
- if there is rhabdomyolysis then alkalinization of urine and mannitol can reduce kidney damage.

- Renal replacement therapy is mainly in the form of continuous venovenous haemofiltration (CVVH). This is an extra-corporeal circulation that uses ultrafiltration to remove water and toxins. **Indications** include:
  - electrolyte disturbance;
  - metabolic acidosis;
  - intoxication with dialysable substances;
  - hypervolaemia;
  - complications from uraemia.
- This system is tolerated well in ITU patients because there are no large changes in intravascular volume associated with intermittent dialysis. However, there is a high risk of sepsis owing to large-bore central venous lines.

NEUROLOGICAL

- Maintenance of blood pressure and oxygenation helps to preserve neurological function.
- Monitoring includes:
  - **Intra-cranial pressure monitoring**.
  - **Jugular bulb oxygen saturation monitoring**:
    - measures the demand by the brain for oxygen.
  - **Transcranial Doppler ultrasound**:
    - monitors cerebral blood flow.
  - **Brain tissue oxygenation**:
    - measures the oxygen pressure.
  - **Electroencephalography**:
    - shows seizures and cerebral activity
  - **Clinical observation**:
    - watching for appropriateness of response in conscious patients. Pupillary reflexes are monitored, but any changes are a late sign.
- Other important physiological parameters to maintain in order to prevent secondary brain injury are:
  - **Blood sugar level**:
    - hyperglycaemia should be avoided with the use of insulin, as it can cause lactic acidosis.
  - **Osmolality and sodium levels**:
    - low osmolality creates a diffusion gradient that can lead to cerebral **oedema**.

Intensive therapy unit/critical care

- **Sedation levels**:
  - restlessness or agitation can cause a sudden rise in the intracranial pressure; sedation is also thought to reduce O_2 metabolism in the brain.
- **Position**:
  - head tilted upwards can help cerebral perfusion pressure, but the MAP must also be maintained.
- **CO_2**:
  - as it is a potent vasodilator in the brain.

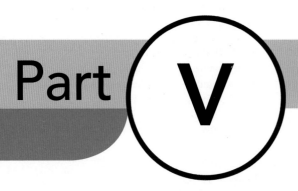

Part V

Self-assessment

Questions

PRE-ASSESSMENT: EMQs

For each of the following questions, please choose the single most likely pre-existing condition responsible for the anaesthetic complications. Each option may be used once, more than once or not at all.

Options:

1) Aortic stenosis.
2) Chronic anaemia.
3) Chronic obstructive pulmonary disease.
4) Diabetes.
5) Hypertension.
6) Renal failure.
7) Rheumatoid arthritis.
8) Sickle cell disease.
9) Unstable angina.
10) Upper respiratory tract infection.

Question 1:

A 70-year-old woman is in the induction room. She has been pre-oxygenated and induced using propofol ready for an operation on a strangulated hernia. She suffers from gastro-oesophageal reflux disease so the decision was made to secure her airway using an endotracheal tube. However, reduced neck mobility makes insertion impossible.

Question 2:

A 58-year-old man has been induced and his anaesthesia is currently being maintained using isoflurane. He is undergoing elective fixation of a fractured radius. After 10 minutes of surgery, the anaesthetic machine monitors show an alarm as he is no longer in sinus rhythm and there are clear ventricular arrhythmias. His blood pressure is also low at 72/40 mmHg. On addition of an inotropic drug, his blood pressure is still low.

Question 3:

A 19-year-old woman is on the ward after an emergency salpingectomy for a ruptured ectopic pregnancy. She is 1 day post-operative and has developed a bacterial pneumonia and is now being treated with antibiotics.

For each of the following questions, please choose the single most likely feature of the history which could have predicted the anaesthetic complication. Each option may be used once, more than once or not at all.

Options:

1) Arrhythmias.
2) Cough.
3) Family history of myocardial infarction.
4) Family history of thromboembolism.
5) Joint pain.
6) Recurrent fits.
7) Shortness of breath.
8) Smokes 40 a day.
9) Weight gain and cold intolerance.
10) Wheeze.

Question 4:

A 52-year-old woman is under anaesthesia for an elective septo-rhinoplasty. Her airway is managed using a laryngeal mask airway with a throat pack to prevent aspiration of blood. She had been given alfentanil to cover the pain. She stopped making any respiratory effort after receiving the drug and has been mechanically ventilated throughout the procedure. At the end of the procedure, the maintenance gas was switched off and the patient ventilated by a bag and mask until she started breathing spontaneously. Even when trying to induce spontaneous breathing by decreasing the respiratory rate and increasing CO_2, it took 15 minutes before she began breathing herself.

Question 5:

A 35-year-old morbidly obese woman is recovering from an anterior bowel resection for an adenocarcinoma. She is 2 days post-operative and has developed shortness of breath and sharp pain on inspiration.

Question 6:

A 63-year-old overweight man is in the induction room for a transurethral resection of the prostate. He is induced using propofol and maintained using isoflurane. After 2 minutes of breathing in isoflurane, his face becomes red, he starts to gag and his eyes start to produce tears.

PRE-ASSESSMENT: SBAs

Question 7:

An 81-year-old man is in the anaesthetic room being prepared for a left hip replacement. He is having a spinal anaesthetic as he has many concurrent medical conditions and the anaesthetist would like to keep him awake throughout the procedure. The spinal needle is inserted and is demonstrated to be in place by a flashback of cerebrospinal fluid, then bupavicaine is administered. However, after insertion, a large haematoma rapidly develops, which takes 2 weeks to settle after a successful operation. Which one of his medications is likely to have caused thc haematoma formation?

1) Digoxin.
2) Doxazosin.
3) Furosemide.
4) Lisinopril.
5) Warfarin.

Question 8:

A 68-year-old male patient is admitted with a gangrenous right foot, which requires a below-knee amputation. He is overweight, has type 1 diabetes and has ischaemic heart disease. He is found to be dehydrated, potassium and sodium deficient and markedly acidotic. The junior doctor caring for him on the ward gives a rapid infusion of normal saline but is unsure of how to proceed further. Which one of the following therapeutic regimes would be the most appropriate for this patient prior to surgery?

1) Insulin.
2) Insulin and dextrose.
3) Insulin, dextrose and potassium.
4) Insulin, dextrose, potassium and magnesium.
5) Insulin, dextrose, potassium, magnesium and bicarbonate.

Question 9:

A 39-year-old woman is admitted for surgery to remove a large ovarian mass on suspicion of malignancy. She is otherwise fit and well and on no medications. She is extremely distressed, as she has a family history of breast cancer and is convinced this will turn out to be malignant. When she is assessed pre-operatively, she inquires about any medications which might be able to calm her nerves. The anaesthetist writes her up for an anxiolytic which can be administered pre-operatively. Which of the following anxiolytics is most likely to be chosen in this scenario?

1) Citalopram.
2) Lorazepam.
3) Midazolam.
4) Propranolol.
5) Temazepam.

Answers

PRE-ASSESSMENT: EMQs

Answer 1:

7) **Rheumatoid arthritis** (RA): this is associated with restricted neck movements and restricted mouth opening because of temporomandibular joint involvement. However, cervical instability can also occur (in around 25% of those with RA), which would make over-extension of the neck very dangerous. Cervical instability is caused by laxity in the atlanto-axial ligaments, which leads to erosion of the odontoid peg. On extension of the neck, it is possible for atlanto-axial subluxation to occur, which could lead to cord compression. A rare complication for patients with RA may be dislocation of the cricoarytenoid joints, which could block the airway. Problems such as this should be identified in pre-assessment.

Answer 2:

1) **Aortic stenosis**: the most common anaesthetic-related complications of aortic stenosis would be ventricular arrhythmias, incipient cardiac failure and a fixed cardiac output. This patient was having arrhythmias and his low blood pressure was unresponsive to inotropic support as his cardiac output was fixed. Aortic stenosis can be shown clinically by an ejection systolic murmur and a radiograph may show a calcified aortic valve. An echocardiograph would be diagnostic and gives a better idea of left ventricular function. A highly stenosed aortic valve requires angioplasty or valve replacement and elective surgery should be avoided because of the high risk of myocardial infarction.

Answer 3:

10) **Upper respiratory tract infection** (URTI): recent or concurrent URTIs are associated with a significantly increased incidence of post-operative chest infection. In this case, this complication was unavoidable because the fact that this patient may have had a URTI would not have prevented her from going into theatre, as an ectopic pregnancy is a surgical emergency. However, in elective patients, the presence of a URTI would mean postponing surgery for 4 weeks at least to prevent this complication.

Answer 4:

9) **Weight gain and cold intolerance**: the symptoms of weight gain and cold intolerance suggest a history of hypothyroidism. Untreated hypothyroidism can cause many different problems during anaesthesia. The problems reported include severe hypotension, cardiac arrest, extreme sensitivity to opioids and

anaesthetic agents, which can lead to respiratory depression and prolonged unconsciousness and hypothyroid coma. This means that patients with symptoms suggestive of hypothyroidism should be investigated pre-operatively (shown by elevated thyroid-stimulating hormone or low free T4). Hypothyroid patients should be effectively treated with thyroxine prior to surgery and be shown to have normal thyroid hormone levels.

Answer 5:

4) **Family history of thromboembolism**: patients with a family history of pulmonary embolism or deep vein thrombosis are at an increased risk of thromboembolism. Additionally, patients who are likely to be immobile for prolonged periods post-operatively are at a greatly increased risk. A venous thromboembolism chart will be filled in pre-operatively, but appropriate management of patients at very high risk should be undertaken.

Answer 6:

8) **Smokes 40 a day**: other appropriate answers to this question would be wheeze, cough and shortness of breath. Any patient with reactive airways, such as asthmatics or those with chronic obstructive pulmonary disease, may have bronchospasm and cough in response to inhaled anaesthetics, especially isoflurane. Heavy smokers (anyone who smokes more than 20 a day) are at risk of increased sputum production, increased reactivity in their airways and atelectasis. Cough or airway irritation in patients under anaesthesia with a controlled airway is likely to manifest as face reddening, tearing and gagging. Smokers should be advised to abstain from smoking for as long as possible prior to surgery, as even 12–24 hours of non-smoking will reduce the amount of carbon monoxide and nicotine in their system. Sevoflurane can be used as an alternative to isoflurane in patients with reactive airways as it is less irritant.

PRE-ASSESSMENT: SBAs

Answer 7:

5) **Warfarin**: many, many patients will be on anti-coagulants such as warfarin. This must be taken into consideration in patients who will be undergoing elective surgery. Warfarin should be stopped 2–4 days prior to surgery but can be reversed rapidly (over 3–6 hours) by administering vitamin K. Heparins (such as clexane) will be reversed only 2–4 hours after stopping the drug.

Answer 8:

3) **Insulin, dextrose and potassium**: the patient should have his blood sugar tested immediately. The addition of low potassium and sodium, dehydration and acidosis should lead to investigation for ketoacidosis, which is a

complication of poorly controlled diabetes. Diabetic ketoacidosis (DKA) can be fatal if not treated and must be reversed prior to surgery. Patients with poorly controlled diabetes present significant problems to the anaesthetist; for example, their stress response to surgery will be impaired and they have a greatly increased risk of myocardial infarction or other end-organ failures. He should be treated initially with aggressive fluid therapy (0.9% saline is fine). Insulin should then be started, with frequent blood sugar monitoring; 5% dextrose should be given, as blood glucose usually falls to low levels; K^+ must be replaced, as its levels will fall further with correction of acidosis. Magnesium excretion can be increased in patients with DKA, but is generally corrected when the patient begins eating and drinking again. Bicarbonate is very rarely given, as the acidosis will be corrected by the other therapies.

Answer 9:

2) Lorazepam: this patient would benefit from anxiolysis as she is likely to be agitated and distressed. Benzodiazepines are usually the drug of choice for anxiolytic premedication. Midazolam is a rapid and short-acting benzodiazepine, which is commonly given during induction to give a relative amnesia and create a smooth induction. It would not be appropriate in this case as it will wear off rapidly. Temazepam is a long-lasting benzodiazepine, with a duration of action of less than 12 hours. This means timing the administration of the drug is vital to achieving anxiolysis that lasts until surgery. This is appropriate in patients who will undergo day surgery, as it will wear off with minimal hangover effect. Lorazepam takes longer to work than temazepam (around 90 minutes) but also has a longer duration, which means timing when it is given can be less precise. It also has some amnesic properties. It is appropriate in this case as the patient will be admitted for several days post-operatively. Propranolol would be indicated in patients with intrusive somatic symptoms to their anxiety. Citalopram is a selective serotonin reuptake inhibitor and not appropriate for premedication.

In the anaesthetic room

Questions

AIRWAY MANAGEMENT: EMQs

For each of the following questions, please choose the single most likely airway adjunct or technique to be used for each patient. Each option may be used once, more than once or not at all.

Options

1) Bag and mask.
2) Endotracheal tube.
3) Guedel airway.
4) Head tilt, chin lift.
5) Jaw thrust.
6) Laryngeal mask airway.
7) Laryngoscope.
8) Nasopharyngeal tube.
9) Throat pack.
10) Tracheostomy.

Question 1:

A 78-year-old woman is found unconscious on the floor in one of the wards and, as a member of the crash team, you rush to see her. As the first to arrive, you aim to assess and secure her airway. There are no signs of blockages in her mouth and she is breathing, so you perform a head tilt and chin lift. Her breathing is noisy and you can hear snoring so you attempt a jaw thrust, which does not stop the noise.

Question 2:

A 24-year-old man is due to undergo surgery for a displaced fractured femur. He has been appropriately starved and has no other concurrent medical problems. He is induced using propofol and midazolam and pre-oxygenated.

Question 3:

A 15-year-old girl is brought in for emergency surgery for acute appendicitis. She is induced using thiopentone, cricoid pressure applied and suxamethonium administered.

For each of the following questions, please choose the single most likely answer for each patient. Each option may be used once, more than once or not at all.

Options

1) Cricothyroidotomy.
2) Fibreoptic laryngoscopy.
3) Grade 1 laryngoscopic view.
4) Grade 2 laryngoscopic view.
5) Grade 3 laryngoscopic view.
6) Mallampati class I.
7) Mallampati class II.
8) Mallampati class III.
9) Mallampati class IV.
10) Tracheostomy.

Question 4:

A 64-year-old man is in the pre-assessment clinic. On assessing the airway, the anaesthetist finds that he is able to see the patient's soft palate only on full mouth opening.

Question 5:

A 59-year-old man is being prepared for surgery to replace a prolapsed mitral valve. He has severe temporomandibular rheumatoid arthritis and is graded Mallampati class IV on airway assessment. The anaesthetist anticipates a very difficult intubation and considers adjuncts.

Question 6:

A 33-year-old woman is brought into the Accident and Emergency Department from a house fire. She has suffered full-thickness burns to the face, trunk and arms. Wheeze is heard on breathing. She requires urgent escharotomy (division of the toughened burnt skin to prevent compartment syndrome). Her airway is obstructed and her saturations dropping. Her airway must be controlled immediately.

Question 7:

A fit and well 72-year-old woman is having elective surgery for a vaginal prolapse. She is pre-oxygenated to 100% and induced using sevoflurane. On laryngoscopy, only her epiglottis is visible.

AIRWAY MANAGEMENT: SBAs

Question 8:

You are the first on the scene at a road traffic collision between an articulated lorry and a small car. The driver of the lorry is clearly distressed but appears to be unharmed. The driver of the car was not wearing a seatbelt and was ejected through the front windscreen onto the road. Traffic is being diverted already, an ambulance has been called and as the only medic at the scene you step in to assess the driver. He is lying on his back on the road, unconscious. His airway is patent, but you can hear a gurgling noise. He is taking shallow and rapid breaths and has a weak pulse. You have no equipment with you but want to secure his airway. Which one of the following would be the most efficient way?

1) Chin lift, jaw thrust.
2) Give rescue breaths.
3) Jaw thrust.
4) Sweep his airway with your fingers.
5) Turn him on his side.

Question 9:

A patient who has been in a fight after a night out comes into the Accident and Emergency Department with severe lacerations to the scalp, broken ribs and a decreased level of consciousness. He has been drinking heavily and thought to have consumed around 15 pints of lager. On examination you find he has some blood in his mouth and is missing some teeth. He is making gurgling noises when he breathes and is tachypnoeic and tachycardic. He is not responding to voice and will not open his eyes, but recoils away when you apply a sternal rub. His pupils react equally to light and there are no signs of focal neurology. On examination of his head you see clear bruising over his mastoid bone and he has two black eyes. You decide to secure his airway; which adjunct would be most appropriate?

1) Endotracheal tube.
2) Guedel airway.
3) Laryngeal mask airway.
4) Nasopharyngeal airway.
5) No intervention.

Answers

AIRWAY MANAGEMENT: EMQs

Answer 1:

3) **Guedel airway:** in the unconscious patient securing the airway is vital. Simple airway manoeuvres such as head tilt and chin lift will help to keep the airway patent. However, to allow you to move quickly and free up your hands, it is a good idea to insert an oropharyngeal airway, such as a Guedel. This will sit over the tongue and prevent it from slipping back and blocking the airway. It is particularly appropriate in this patient as snoring sounds often indicate a

degree of airway blockage by the soft palate. Guedel airways must be measured properly (from incisors to angle of the jaw). A small airway is useless as it will not depress the tongue and a large one will block the airway.

Answer 2:

6) **Laryngeal mask airway (LMA):** an LMA would be appropriate in this patient, as he is not at risk of aspirating gastric contents and has been appropriately starved. An LMA allows easy and fast insertion. Inserting an endotracheal tube would also be reasonable, but is often not quite as easy or quick to insert.

Answer 3:

2) **Endotracheal tube:** this patient has not been starved and is therefore at risk of aspirating gastric contents. A laryngeal mask airway or nasopharyngeal airway will not allow complete protection against aspiration. The endotracheal tube has an inflatable cuff that sits around the trachea and prevents any aspirated contents from entering the trachea. Suction will be necessary when extubating and the patient can be positioned on her side.

Answer 4:

9) **Mallampati class IV:** Mallampati grading is used when assessing airways to help predict a difficult intubation. The higher the grading, the more difficult the intubation is assumed to be. For more information on Mallampati grading, see Chapter 2, Preparing for surgery.

Answer 5:

2) **Fibreoptic laryngoscopy:** in a patient who displays signs of a potentially difficult intubation, additional techniques should be considered prior to the induction. Fibreoptic laryngoscopy can be used in patients with anticipated severely difficult intubation but without airway obstruction. Severe reduction of head and neck movements may indicate fibreoptic laryngoscopy to ensure that tracheal intubation is successful.

Answer 6:

1) **Cricothyroidotomy:** patients who have severe airway obstruction and deteriorating clinical state may require urgent cricothyroidotomy, under local anaesthesia. Tracheostomy is slower than cricothyroidotomy, so would be used in an emergency situation. Burns patients are at high risk of airway damage owing to smoke inhalation and an assessment of their airway should be undertaken immediately.

Answer 7:

5) Grade 3 laryngoscopic view: the view at laryngoscopy is graded according to the visibility of the vocal cords and epiglottis. The pharyngeal view (Mallampati score) gives a guide to the probable laryngoscopic view. Details of laryngoscopic grading can be found in Chapter 4, Airways and ventilation.

AIRWAY MANAGEMENT: SBAs

Answer 8:

3) Jaw thrust: the chin lift and jaw thrust manoeuvres are an effective way of keeping a patient's airway open. This patient has quite possibly suffered a C-spine injury, so should not be moved. This includes a head tilt. Sweeping a patient's mouth should only be done if a blockage can be seen, or you risk pushing something further in. Rescue breaths are not appropriate in a patient who is spontaneously breathing and are no longer recommended in the most recent basic life support guidelines.

Answer 9:

4) Endotracheal tube: from the description in the question, this man's Glasgow Coma Scale (GCS) score is 6 (eye response, 1; verbal response, 1; motor response, 4) and his airway is clearly at risk. He should be immediately induced with a rapid sequence and intubated to secure his airway. When considering airway management in patients with a head injury, base of skull fracture must be excluded. In this example, the patient has incurred a head injury severe enough to reduce his GCS score. He also has classic signs of a base of skull fracture, such as mastoid bruising (commonly known as Battle's sign) and panda eyes. Insertion of a nasopharyngeal airway is absolutely contra-indicated because of the risk of perforation through the skull into the brain.

16 Practice of anaesthesia

Questions

MAINTENANCE OF ANAESTHESIA: EMQs

For each of the following questions, please choose the single most likely anaesthetic agent to be used as anaesthetic maintenance for each patient. Each option may be used once, more than once or not at all.

Options

1) Adrenaline.
2) Atracurium.
3) Fentanyl.
4) Halothane.
5) Isoflurane.

6) Morphine.
7) Propofol.
8) Sevoflurane.
9) Suxamethonium.
10) Thiopental.

Question 1:

An 11-year-old asthmatic patient is induced using propofol for bilateral insertion of grommets.

Question 2:

A 55-year-old woman is on the intensive therapy unit (ITU) with bacterial endocarditis and disseminated intravascular coagulopathy. She is being kept lightly anaesthetized and mechanically ventilated with multisystem support while in ITU.

Question 3:

A 39-year-old has surgery to drain a pilonidal abscess. She is otherwise fit and well, with no previous medical history of note and is a non-smoker. She is induced using propofol and midazolam.

MAINTENANCE OF ANAESTHESIA: SBAs

Question 4:

A 69-year-old man who was rushed to hospital for repair of a leaking abdominal aortic aneurysm is induced using thiopental and cricoid pressure. Suxamethonium is given and muscle fasciculations are seen after 30 seconds. A good level of neuromuscular blockade is achieved. What one of the following anaesthetic agents should be used to maintain this man's anaesthesia?

1) Isoflurane.
2) Nitrous oxide.
3) Propofol.
4) Sevoflurane.
5) Thiopental.

GENERAL ANAESTHESIA: EMQs

For each of the following questions, please choose the single most likely agent to be used for the type of procedure described. Each option may be used once, more than once, or not at all.

Options

1) Halothane.
2) Isoflurane.
3) Ketamine.
4) Midazolam.
5) Nitrous oxide.
6) Propofol.
7) Remifentanil.
8) Sevoflurane.
9) Suxamethonium.
10) Thiopental.

Question 5:

A 2-year-old girl is due for induction of planned surgery to correct congenital talipes equinovarus. She has no other medical history of note and is otherwise fit and well. Which induction agent should be used?

Question 6:

A 45-year-old man with severe depression requires sedation for electroconvulsive therapy. He has no previous medical history and is otherwise fit and well. Which other drug would be used apart from the anaesthetic agent?

Question 7:

A patient who underwent routine surgery yesterday complains to her nurse that she felt pain when she was given the anaesthetic injection that put her to sleep. Which inducing agent was this?

FLUID: EMQs

For each of the following questions, please choose the single most appropriate fluid to administer. Answers may be used once, more than once or not at all.

Options

1) 0.45% saline.
2) 0.9% saline.
3) 0.9% saline + 40 mmol of KCl.
4) 5% albumin.
5) 5% dextrose.
6) 5% dextrose + 40 mmol of KCl.
7) 20% dextrose.
8) Gelofusine.
9) Hartmann's solution.
10) Packed red blood cells.

Question 8:

A 25-year old man who is a known type 1 diabetic is admitted with lethargy, vomiting and acetone breath. His blood glucose level is 27 mmol/L, there are ketones on dipstick and his potassium is 5.9 mmol/L.

Question 9:

An 89-year-old man who went to a reunion dinner last week is admitted with a 4 day history of diarrhoea and vomiting. On examination he is clinically dehydrated. His urea and electrolyte levels show Na^+ of 150 mmol/L, K^+ of 4.5 mmol/L, urea of 17.1 mmol/L and creatinine of 280 mmol/L.

Question 10:

A 35-year-old patient with a known history of alcohol excess who was admitted with ascites, jaundice and lethargy is on the gastroenterology ward. He starts to vomit fresh blood, his blood pressure decreases and he becomes tachycardic.

Question 11:

A 59-year-old patient with insulin-dependent diabetes is found on the ward after large bowel resection with a decreased level of consciousness and confusion. He is haemodynamically stable.

Question 12:

A 56-year-old man with poorly controlled diabetes on oral medications is found to have a potassium level of 2.3 mmol/L after being treated with intravenous furosemide for pulmonary oedema.

Question 13:

A 56-year-old woman who has been admitted for a cholecystectomy is found to have a low blood pressure on routine observations; you notice that her blood pressure has been dropping throughout the day and she is now spiking a temperature to 39.4°C.

FLUID: SBAs

Question 14:

A 45-year-old man on an upper gastrointestinal ward, who was admitted for decompensated liver failure, begins to complain of passing black motions. On further questioning he admits that he has been passing these motions all day. You notice that his blood pressure has been deteriorating throughout the day. Which one of the following would be an inappropriate fluid to administer?
1) 5% dextrose.
2) Gelofusine.
3) Hartmann's solution.
4) Packed red blood cells.
5) Volplex.

Question 15:

A junior doctor on the wards wants to administer Hartmann's solution to a 64 year old man who has had a transurethral resection of his prostate. Which of these electrolytes is not present in Hartmann's solution?
1) Bicarbonate.
2) Calcium.
3) Chloride.
4) Magnesium.
5) Potassium.

ELECTROLYTES: EMQs

For each of the following questions, please choose the correct electrolyte imbalance to explain the presenting complaint. Answers may be used once, more than once or not at all.

Options

1) Hypercalcaemia.
2) Hyperkalaemia.
3) Hypermagnesaemia.
4) Hyponatraemia.
5) Hypophosphataemia.

6) Hypocalcaemia.
7) Hypokalaemia.
8) Hypomagnesaemia.
9) Hypernatraemia.
10) Hyperphosphataemia.

Question 16:

A 68-year-old woman who has been a lifelong smoker presents to the 2-week-wait clinic with weight loss, cough and haemoptysis. On taking the history the doctor finds that that she has been suffering from confusion lately along with nausea, vomiting and visual disturbances.

Question 17:

A 67-year-old man presents to the urology clinic to be seen about problems he has been having with frequency, nocturia, hesitancy and poor flow. He also admits to having lower back pain and his wife says he has been having abdominal pain and changes in mood recently.

Question 18:

A 56-year-old man who has recently been diagnosed with acute myeloid leukaemia and started on combination chemotherapy presents to his GP complaining of muscle spasm; on examination the GP is able to elicit Chvostek's sign.

ECG: SBAs

Question 19:

A 30-year-old woman attends pre-assessment clinic for an elective cholecys-tectomy for recurrent gallstones. She mentions that she has suffered from bulimia nervosa for much of her life, which has been worse recently because of severe stress at work. She is found to have the ECG shown in Fig. 16.1.

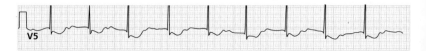

Fig. 16.1 Lead V5 of 12-lead ECG.

Which of the following electrolyte abnormalities is most likely to cause this picture?
1) Hypercalcaemia.
2) Hyperkalaemia.
3) Hypocalcaemia.
4) Hypokalaemia.
5) Hyponatraemia.

Question 20:

A 30-year-old woman who has been on the burns unit for 2 days after suffering 60% partial thickness burns complains of tingling in her fingers and around her mouth, as well as some muscle cramps. She is found to have the ECG shown in Fig. 16.2.

Answer 5:

5) **Ketamine**: the dissociative anaesthetic ketamine can be used intramuscularly in paediatric patients if intravenous access cannot be obtained and the patient is unlikely to tolerate an inhaled induction agent. It is avoided in adult patients because of its tendency to cause hallucinations and nightmares, but the incidence of this is much lower in children.

Answer 6:

8) **Propofol**: this is by far the most commonly used induction agent because of its rapid action, side-effect profile and relative safety.

Answer 7:

5) **Rapid sequence induction**: this appendicitis patient has an acute abdomen and he needs an urgent operation. We do not know when he last had food but gastric emptying will be delayed even if there is no ileus. Therefore, the risk of regurgitation and subsequent aspiration is high. To protect his airway an endotracheal tube must be secured following a rapid sequence induction.

Answer 8:

1) **Bier's block**: a woman who recently had an inferior myocardial infarct is a high-risk patient and alternatives to general anaesthesia should be considered. A Bier's block (intravenous regional anaesthesia) can provide anaesthesia for minor surgery to the distal ends of both upper and lower limbs. A tourniquet is applied and a suitable local anaesthetic injected intravenously. A double cuff can reduce discomfort. A subclavian perivascular block is contraindicated in day case surgery because of the risk of pneumothorax and in anti-coagulated patients.

Answer 9:

1) **Spinal anaesthesia**: a regional block is safer in this patient with multiple co-morbidities.

Answer 10:

1) **14G cannula**: a pregnant woman undergoing an emergency caesarean section is at risk of blood loss, but needs rapid intravenous access. Fortunately, because of her hypervolaemic state, intravenous cannulation with very large-bore needles in each antecubital fossa is an easy task in the hands of a skilled anaesthetist.

Answer 11:

7) **Central venous line**: a patient undergoing very invasive major surgery will need a central venous line both for delivery of fluids and drugs and for central venous pressure monitoring. They will also be cannulated peripherally.

Self-assessment

Answer 12:

3) 18G cannula: in this fit and healthy individual, in whom there is little risk of major blood loss or complications, a relatively small gauge intravenous cannula will suffice. A 20G would also be acceptable.

INDUCTION OF ANAESTHESIA: SBAs

Answer 13:

3) General anaesthetic, laryngeal mask airway and spontaneous ventilation: this woman is a good candidate for general anaesthesia. She will not need muscle paralysis for this operation and is at low risk of aspiration so a laryngeal mask airway will be an effective airway. This operation could not be performed under local anaesthetic because of the wound size, location and presence of infection. Regional anaesthesia could be used, but in this patient represents a higher risk of complications than general anaesthetic (GA). However, GA could be justified as the surgeons may find they need to debride through the entire abdominal wall thickness.

18

On the wards

Questions

PAIN MANAGEMENT: EMQs

For each of the following questions, please select the most appropriate analgesic agent to be used.

Options

1) Amitriptyline.	6) Ibuprofen.
2) Co-codamol.	7) Lidocaine.
3) Dihydrocodeine.	8) Mefenamic acid.
4) Entonox.	9) Morphine.
5) Fentanyl.	10) Naloxone.

Question 1:

A 60-year-old man with inoperable metastatic anorectal cancer is suffering from severe pelvic pain. He is currently taking paracetamol, a non-steroidal anti-inflammatory drug and a weak opiate. What agent can be used to improve the patient's pain relief?

Question 2:

A 56-year-old man has pain in the area where he recently had an acute attack of shingles. In addition to co-codamol and ibuprofen, what could be given to ease his pain?

Question 3:

A 70-year-old man recently diagnosed with prostate cancer has been experiencing moderate dull pain in his middle lower back for 3 weeks. What would be the most effective analgesic agent for his pain?

For each of the following questions, please select the analgesic agent being referred to.

Options

1) Co-codamol.	6) Ibuprofen.
2) Dihydrocodeine.	7) Lidocaine.
3) Entonox.	8) Mefenamic acid.
4) Fentanyl.	9) Morphine.
5) Gabapentin.	10) Naloxone.

Question 4:

This painkiller is particularly effective for treating menstrual pain.

Question 5:

This analgesic agent is sometimes used in special preparations for severe chronic pain uncontrolled by other strong painkillers.

Question 6:

This anti-epileptic drug can be used as an adjunct for neuropathic pain.

For each of the following questions, please select the analgesic agent being referred to:

Options

1) Buprenorphine.	6) Morphine sulphate.
2) Codeine.	7) Oxycodone.
3) Diclofenac.	8) Paracetamol.
4) Fentanyl.	9) Pethidine.
5) Ibuprofen.	10) Tramadol.

Question 7:

Used for breakthrough pain in patients already receiving opioid therapy for chronic pain. Commonly applied in a patch form. A World Health Organization class 3 analgesic.

Question 8:

A World Health Organization class 1 analgesic that is converted to a toxic metabolite, N-acetyl-p-benzoquinoneimine, which is inactivated by conjugation to reduced glutathione.

Question 9:

A World Health Organization class 3 analgesic that produces analgesia by two mechanisms, an opioid effect and an enhancement of serotonergic and adrenergic pathways.

SEPSIS: EMQs

Please select the most appropriate answer for each of the following questions.

Options

1) Call for senior help.
2) Check airways.
3) Check breathing.
4) Check circulation.
5) Give 6 litres O_2 via simple mask.
6) Give 15 litres O_2 via non-rebreathe mask.
7) Give antibiotics empirically.
8) Give a fluid challenge.
9) Obtain intravenous access.
10) Take septic screen.

You are the junior doctor called to see a 68-year-old woman who has become acutely unwell over the last few hours. She is 8 days post-oesophagectomy for an oesophageal carcinoma. When you see her she appears unwell, pale, blue around the lips and out of breath, but asks you to help her.

Question 10:

What do you do next?

Question 11:

Her lips look less blue, her saturations are 96% on ~60% oxygen and her respiratory rate has slowed to 22 breaths/min. Her blood pressure is 90/46 mmHg and heart rate is 98 beats/min. What do you do now?

Question 12:

Now with help, you have managed to get the patient to be haemodynamically stable. Auscultation of her chest reveals coarse crackles in the left upper zone. What do you do now?

For each of the following questions, please select the most appropriate answer.

Options

1) Acute kidney injury.
2) Chronic renal failure.
3) Gastroenteritis.
4) Lobar pneumonia.
5) Peritonitis.
6) Pyelonephritis.

7) Sepsis.
8) Septic shock.

9) Severe sepsis.
10) Urinary tract infection.

A 55-year-old man is on a surgical ward 6 days following anterior resection for Dukes A carcinoma. You are the on-call house officer and are called to see him by one of the nurses. Assessment reveals the following: A – airways patent; B – breathing spontaneously, respiratory rate 23 breaths/min, saturations 98% on 28% O_2, chest clear; C – peripherally cool, capillary refill time 4 seconds, pulse 112 beats/min, blood pressure 100/72 mmHg; D – drowsy, Glasgow Coma Scale score 13. His temperature has been fluctuating over the last 6 hours and his abdomen is very tender.

Question 13:
What condition is the patient suffering from that can be deduced from the information above?

Question 14:
A few hours later, during which the patient has been receiving fluids and antibiotics, blood results return showing raised urea and raised creatinine, which has more than doubled since the last test 12 hours ago. His urine output has been steadily dropping over the last 4 hours. What complication has developed?

Question 15:
What can you now diagnose this patient with?

For each of the following questions, please select the most appropriate answer.

Options

1) 0.45% saline.
2) 0.9% saline.
3) 5% dextrose solution.
4) 50% glucose.
5) Dextrose–saline.
6) Fresh frozen plasma and platelets.

7) Hartmann's solution.
8) Hydroxyethyl starch colloid solution.
9) O-negative whole blood.
10) Packed red cells.

Question 16:
When administering a fluid challenge to a hypotensive septic patient, which crystalloid fluid do you not use?

Question 17:
Which fluid will provide the greatest increase in intravascular volume?

Question 18:

A patient develops disseminated intravascular coaogulopathy as a complication of septic shock. What intravenous infusion can be given to reduce the chance of haemorrhage?

For each of the following questions, please select the most appropriate therapy.

Options

1) Dexamethasone.	6) Glucagon.
2) Digoxin.	7) Labetalol.
3) Diltiazem.	8) Noradrenaline.
4) Dobutamine.	9) Oxygen.
5) Fluid therapy.	10) Theophylline.

A 58-year-old man is admitted to the intensive therapy unit with severe sepsis following an anastomotic leak after a resection for a Dukes A carcinoma. He is unconscious and is intubated and ventilated.

Question 19:

The patient is noted to have a blood pressure of 70/48 mmHg and pulse of 128 beats/min, sinus rhythm.

Question 20:

The patient's skin is pale and clammy and the capillary refill time is less than 2 seconds but the blood pressure remains low and pulse high. The intensivists decide to try a drug to elevate the blood pressure.

Question 21:

The blood pressure improves to around 110/70 mmHg. However, it is noted that the patient's urine output has been falling and he has been anuric for 3 hours. In addition, blood results return showing deranged liver function tests. A drug is used to attempt to improve organ perfusion.

VOLATILE GASES: EMQs

For each of the following questions, please select the most appropriate answer(s).

Options

1) Desflurane.	4) Halothane.
2) Enflurane.	5) Isoflurane.
3) Ether.	6) Methoxyflurane.

7) Nitrous oxide.
8) Propofol.

9) Sevoflurane.
10) Trichloroethylene (Trilene).

Question 22:
Which inhaled agent is the most potent trigger of malignant hypertension?

Question 23:
Which inhaled agent is not a trigger of malignant hypertension?

Question 24:
Which inhaled agent has the most serious hepatotoxicity?

For each of the following questions, please select the most appropriate answer.

Options

1) Desflurane.	6) Methoxyflurane.
2) Enflurane.	7) Nitrous oxide.
3) Ether.	8) Propofol.
4) Halothane.	9) Sevoflurane.
5) Isoflurane.	10) Trichloroethylene (Trilene).

Question 25:
Which inhaled agent works and wears off the quickest?

Question 26:
Which inhaled agent has the highest minimum alveolar concentration?

Question 27:
Which inhaled agent is preferred for mask induction?

REGIONAL ANAESTHESIA: SBAs

Question 28:
A 66-year-old man is listed for a left inguinal hernia repair to be done under a spinal anaesthetic. What layers will the needle pass through in order from most superficial to most deep?
1) Dura mater, ligamentum flavum, interspinous ligament, supraspinous ligament.
2) Ligamentum flavum, supraspinous ligament, interspinous ligament, dura mater.
3) Supraspinous ligament, interspinous ligament, dura mater, ligamentum flavum.

4) Supraspinous ligament, interspinous ligament, ligamentum flavum, dura mater.

5) Supraspinous ligament, ligamentum flavum, interspinous ligament, dura mater.

REGIONAL ANAESTHESIA: EMQs

For each of the following questions, please choose the single most likely drug responsible. Each option may be used once, more than once or not at all.

Options

1) Adrenaline.
2) Amethocaine.
3) Bupivacaine.
4) Cocaine.
5) Fentanyl.
6) Lidocaine.
7) Lorazepam.
8) Morphine.
9) Neostigmine.
10) Ropivacaine.

Question 29:

Often used in ear–nose–throat surgery as it vasoconstricts and so reduces blood loss.

Question 30:

Available as a gel for a topical anaesthetic often used for pre-cannulation in paediatrics.

Question 31:

Given with adrenaline to a patient having excision of a sebaceous cyst under local anaesthetic as a day case.

PRE-OPERATIVE MEDICATIONS: EMQs

For each of the following questions, please choose the single most likely drug. Each option may be used once, more than once or not at all.

Options

1) Atenolol.
2) Cyclizine.
3) Fentanyl.
4) Glycopyrrolate.
5) Metoclopramide.
6) Morphine.
7) Omeprazole.
8) Ondansetron.
9) Ranitidine.
10) Temazepam.

Question 32:

A well-absorbed drug given pre-operatively to relax the patient and cause mild amnesia and sedation.

Question 33:

A prokinetic anti-emetic.

Question 34:

This drug antagonizes $5HT_3$ receptors.

Answers

PAIN MANAGEMENT: EMQs

Answer 1:

9) Morphine: this man has reached level 3 of the World Health Organization guide to managing cancer pain and should be prescribed a strong opioid as his pain is not controlled on weak opioids. Morphine is the first-line strong opioid.

Answer 2:

1) Amitriptyline: this man is suffering from post-herpetic neuralgia. Amitriptyline is a tricyclic anti-depressant drug that can be used as an analgesic adjunct as it is effective at easing neuralgia in addition to its actions on depression. However, it can take 2 or more weeks to become effective.

Answer 3:

6) Ibuprofen: this man is likely to be suffering from the pain associated with bony metastases. Non-steroidal anti-inflammatory drugs (NSAIDs) are the most effective analgesic agents for bony pain but it is important that it is only prescribed for this man if there are no contraindications – renal function should be thoroughly assessed before starting NSAIDs in elderly patients. In addition, this man would need investigating for his potential metastases.

Answer 4:

8) Mefenamic acid: this non-steroidal anti-inflammatory drug is effective in treating menstrual pain as it reduces inflammation and uterine contractions by an unknown mechanism.

Answer 5:

4) Fentanyl: this is a very powerful (approximately $100 \times$ the potency of morphine) semi-synthetic opioid with strong agonistic action at the μ-opioid receptors. It can be used to treat patients with chronic pain in the form of slow-release transdermal patches and also in the form of quick-acting lozenges, 'lollipops', nasal sprays and inhalers that can be used to counteract 'breakthrough pain'.

Answer 6:

5) Gabapentin: although not licensed for this indication, gabapentin has been shown to be an effective treatment for neuropathic pain, migraine headache and nystagmus, in addition to its anti-epileptic actions.

Answer 7:

4) Fentanyl: this is a transdermal strong synthetic opioid. Produced in a patch which sticks to the skin, it releases fentanyl over 72 hours. After this time it should be replaced.

Answer 8:

8) Paracetamol: a simple analgesic, which is used first line. It works alongside stronger analgesics, reducing their required dose.

Answer 9:

10) Tramadol: useful in moderate pain, and can be given alongside paracetamol and morphine. Tramadol is a useful alternative to codeine phosphate, a drug also in class 3 of the World Health Organization scale, as it only rarely causes constipation.

SEPSIS: EMQs

Answer 10:

6) Give 15 litres O_2 via non-rebreather mask: this woman is clearly acutely unwell. Following the ABC approach: by speaking to you she has demonstrated airway patency. However, she appears cyanotic and out of breath despite having oxygen via nasal cannula. You should treat as soon as you find a problem; in this case by giving as much oxygen as is possible.

Answer 11:

8) Give a fluid challenge: again, following the ABC approach, you should treat as soon as you find a problem; in this case the apparent hypovolaemia. You also need to call for help, as this woman is very unwell.

Self-assessment

Answer 12:

10) Take septic screen: clinically, the patient has sepsis as a result of a likely lobar pneumonia. She needs antibiotics as soon as possible, and these should not be delayed. However, before they are given, blood and swabs should be taken for culture and sensitivity, to allow more directed antibiotic therapy.

Answer 13:

7) Sepsis: the patient has more than two criteria for the systemic inflammatory response syndrome (respiratory rate > 20 breaths/min, heart rate > 90 beats/min, abnormal temperature) in the presence of suspected infection. Therefore sepsis can be diagnosed.

Answer 14:

1) Acute kidney injury: oliguria, raised urea and raised creatinine suggest acute kidney injury. Using the RIFLE criteria (see Chapter 8, In the operating theatre) this is graded as injury (I) as the creatinine has doubled over 12 hours.

Answer 15:

9) Severe sepsis: acute kidney injury demonstrates organ dysfunction, which means the patient now has severe sepsis. As his blood pressure is in the normal range, his kidney injury is unlikely to be caused by septic shock.

Answer 16:

3) 5% dextrose solution: the glucose in dextrose solution is rapidly absorbed from the bloodstream, and once the glucose, which is responsible for the fluid's osmolality, is absorbed the fluid is soon redistributed to the extra-vascular space. For this reason, dextrose provides only a very transient improvement in blood pressure, if any. All other fluids have been shown to have similar efficacy, although the 'crystalloid vs colloid debate' rages on.

Answer 17:

8) Hydroxyethyl starch colloid solution: colloid solutions (often called plasma expanders) contain very large molecules which cannot move out of the intravascular space. This means that all of the fluid remains in the bloodstream until the molecules are eventually broken down. As sodium chloride can move into the interstitial space, about two-thirds of saline solutions are redistributed out of the intravascular space.

Answer 18:

6) Fresh frozen plasma and platelets: in disseminated intravascular coagulopathy, deranged clotting leads to the consumption of platelets and clotting factors, which may result in haemorrhage. Fresh frozen plasma contains clotting factors and can be used to reduce bleeding in this very serious and often fatal condition. Platelet transfusions and cryoprecipitate (to provide fibrinogen) may also be employed.

Answer 19:

5) **Fluid therapy**: the first intervention to counteract hypotension should be intravenous fluids, crystalloid or colloid, but not dextrose.

Answer 20:

8) **Noradrenaline**: if the patient seems adequately intravascularly filled but blood pressure remains low, the patient has inadequate myocardial function and/or a degree of vasodilation which fluid therapy alone cannot overcome. In this situation an agent with vasopressor (adrenoreceptor agonist) properties, such as noradrenaline (norepinephrine), is appropriate.

Answer 21:

4) **Dobutamine**: if the patient has signs of poor organ perfusion, is cool peripherally (a large core to peripheral temperature difference) and/or has low blood pressure then an agent with more positive inotropic properties is the most appropriate. Adrenaline (epinephrine), dopamine and dobutamine are examples of positive inotropes.

VOLATILE GASES: EMQs

Answer 22:

4) **Halothane**: this is a potent trigger of the rare but life-threatening condition malignant hyperthermia. However, all volatile anaesthetics can potentially trigger malignant hypertension in susceptible individuals. Halothane is no longer available for use in the UK.

Answer 23:

7) **Nitrous oxide**: while not strictly a volatile anaesthetic agent (as it is a vapour at room temperature and a gas at body temperature), nitrous oxide will not trigger malignant hyperthermia.

Answer 24:

4) **Halothane and** 6) **Methoxyflurane**: while all volatile agents affect the liver, halothane is often avoided becaue of potential severe hepatotoxicity. Two types of halothane hepatotoxicity have been observed: type 1, a mild, self-limiting post-operative hepatotoxicity affecting ~20% of patients, and type 2, a rare but potentially fatal hepatitis. Methoxyflurane also causes liver failure.

Answer 25:

1) **Desflurane**: this has an extremely low blood solubility that is responsible for the very rapid onset and offset of its actions. However, its low potency, pungency and high cost prohibit wider use.

Answer 26:

7) **Nitrous oxide**: this has a minimum alveolar concentration of 104, meaning that, at 1 atmostphere pressure, a concentration of 104% nitrous oxide would be necessary to prevent a reaction to a surgical stimulus in 50% of patients. As a concentration of 104% is impossible, the only way to fully anaesthetize a patient with nitrous oxide is to use a hyperbaric chamber. Nitrous oxide is often used in conjunction with another inhaled agent.

Answer 27:

4) **Sevoflurane**: this has a sweet smell, low irritability and has the second fastest onset and offset of volatile anaesthetics after desflurane. For this reason it is the agent most often used for induction.

REGIONAL ANAESTHESIA: SBAs

Answer 28:

4) **Supraspinous ligament, interspinous ligament, ligamentum flavum, dura mater**: see Fig. 6.1 for spinal anatomy.

REGIONAL ANAESTHESIA: EMQs

Answer 29:

2) **Cocaine**: its dual action of local anaesthetic and vasconstrictor is especially useful in rhinoplasties as the nose is highly vascular. Other local anaesthetics, such as lidocaine, do not have such vasoconstriction properties and are therefore mixed with adrenaline.

Answer 30:

2) **Amethocaine**: a local anaesthetic in the ester group.

Answer 31:

6) **Lidocaine**: most commonly used local anaesthetic, given via subcutaneous injection.

PRE-OPERATIVE MEDICATIONS: EMQs

Answer 32:

10) **Temazepam**: this is a benzodiazepine that is rapidly absorbed from the gastrointestinal tract, and therefore is useful pre-operatively as it is fast-acting. Benzodiazepines have a selective action on the limbic system and cerebral cortex – areas that control state of arousal. Diazepam and chlordiazepoxide are long-acting and therefore most useful as anxiolytics, whereas temazepam is short-acting and therefore used as a hypnotic.

Answer 33:

5) **Metoclopramide**: belonging to the benzamine class of drugs, metoclopramide is a central dopamine (D_2) antagonist which increases gastric motility. It is therefore useful in gastrointestinal (GI) causes of nausea and vomiting, but should be avoided in GI obstruction.

Answer 34:

8) **Ondansetron**: an anti-emetic which antagonizes serotonin at $5HT_3$ receptors. Its exact mode of action is unclear, but it has both peripheral and central actions. Previously restricted to use in the control of nausea and vomiting caused by chemo- and radiotherapy because of cost, it is now available as a generic drug. Side-effects include constipation, headache and flushing.

19

Resuscitation and emergencies

Questions

INTRA-OPERATIVE EMERGENCIES: SBA

Question 1:

A 45-year-old obese patient is listed for a right-sided knee arthroplasty; 20 minutes into the operation she becomes hypoxic, saturating at 88%. Her blood pressure is recorded at 85/45 mmHg. On auscultation of the chest, there is a diffuse wheeze throughout and on exposure she has a rash. What is the first thing that should be done when managing this intra-operative complication?
1) Chlorpheniramine.
2) Intravenous fluids.
3) Oxygen.
4) Salbutamol.
5) Stop all likely precipitants.

MUSCLE RELAXANTS: EMQs

From the list below select the most appropriate drug in the following scenarios. Each option may be used once, more than once or not at all.

Options

1) Atracurium.
2) Diamorphine.
3) Diazepam.
4) Diclofenac.
5) Etomidate.

6) Fentanyl.
7) Pancuronium.
8) Propofol.
9) Suxamethonium.
10) Thiopentone.

Question 2:

A healthy woman is scheduled for a laparoscopic sterilization. Which drug will provide suitable muscle relaxation?

Question 3:

A young man is due to have a large lipoma excised from his forearm. Which agent would be a suitable intravenous induction agent to allow placement of a laryngeal mask airway?

Question 4:

A 64 year old man presents for a cystoscopy. A hiatus hernia was diagnosed 6 months ago. His current medication is gaviscon and he has been nil by mouth since midnight. Select a suitable muscle relaxant to allow placement of the endotracheal tube.

ADVANCED LIFE SUPPORT: EMQs

For each of the following questions, please select the most appropriate immediate treatment or action from the list below. Each option may be used once, more than once or not at all.

Options

1) Adenosine.
2) Amiodarone.
3) Basic life support.
4) Call the cardiac arrest team.
5) Check for a central pulse.
6) Defibrillation.
7) Give precordial thump.
8) Lidocaine.
9) Needle decompression.
10) Synchronized DC cardioversion.

Question 5:

A 64-year-old woman who, 10 days ago, had a total hip replacement is found unconscious in the ward toilet. She is unresponsive, apnoeic and pulseless.

Question 6:

A 51-year-old man is in ventricular fibrillation. He has received three defibrillatory shocks and 1 mg of adrenaline intravenously. Two minutes of cardiopulmonary resuscitation is ongoing.

Question 7:

An elderly woman has arrested during the insertion of a right subclavian central line. Adrenaline has been given and 3 minutes of basic life support is ongoing. As the cardiac arrest team leader you notice that the trachea is deviated to the left.

For each of the following questions, please select the most appropriate answer from the list below. Each option may be used once, more than once or not at all.

Options

1) 30:2.
2) Atrial fibrilliation.
3) Atrial flutter.
4) Pulseless electrical activity.
5) Pulseless ventricular tachycardia.
6) Re-entry tachycardia.
7) Respiratory arrest.
8) Sinus bradycardia.
9) Sinus tachycardia.
10) Third-degree heart block.

Question 8:

A non-shockable rhythm seen in cardiac arrest.

Question 9:

A rhythm that can respond to defibrillation in cardiac arrest management.

Question 10:

Organized cardiac electrical activity in the absence of any palpable pulses.

ADVANCED LIFE SUPPORT: SBAs

Question 11:

You arrive at the bedside 5 minutes after the cardiac arrest of a 76-year-old man admitted with shortness of breath and exacerbation of chronic obstructive pulmonary disease. A cannula is in place and there is no pulse. The cardiac monitor shows asystole. Two of your colleagues are performing cardiopulmonary resuscitation at a rate of 30:2. Which one of the following should be the next course of action?

1) Adrenaline 1 mg intramuscularly.
2) Adrenaline 1 mg intravenously.
3) Call for help.
4) Delivery of 150 J biphasic shock.
5) Delivery of a 360 J monophasic shock.

Answers

INTRA-OPERATIVE EMERGENCIES: SBAs

Answer 1:

5) **Stop all likely precipitants**: this describes a case of intra-operative anaphylactic shock, characterized by a drop in blood pressure, wheeze and rash. All actions will be futile before precipitants of the anaphylaxis are stopped. Oxygen should be applied early to reverse any hypoxia.

MUSCLE RELAXANTS: EMQs

Answer 2:

1) **Atracurium**: muscle relaxation is required during the creation of a pneumoperitoneum, which provides a clear view and access to the fallopian tubes. The anticipated duration of surgery is 20–30 minutes, thus atracurium is the best choice. Suxamethonium is too short-acting and pancuronium lasts too long.

Answer 3:

8) **Propofol**: this is the best induction agent when planning to use a laryngeal mask airway. It inhibits the pharyngeal and laryngeal reflexes faster than other agents, providing optimal conditions for inserting the device.

Answer 4:

9) **Suxamethonium**: patients with a hiatus hernia must have their airway protected as quickly as possible following induction of anaesthesia. Failure to protect the airway with an endotracheal tube may lead to aspiration. Suxamethonium is the correct choice as it provides optimum intubating conditions in 30–45 seconds.

ADVANCED LIFE SUPPORT: EMQs

Answer 5:

4) **Call the cardiac arrest team**: this patient has no respiratory or cardiovascular effort. She is therefore in cardiorespiratory arrest and the help of the cardiac arrest team is needed urgently.

Answer 6:

2) Amiodarone: this is the drug given after the fourth cycle of cardiopulmonary resuscitation in shockable cardiac arrests.

Answer 7:

9) Needle decompression: the central line has been misdirected and caused a tension pneumothorax, deviating the mediastinum and causing pressure in the heart leading to decreased cardiac output and ultimately cardiac arrest. Needle decompression of the tension pneumothorax will allow air to escape the thorax and decrease the pressure on the heart. Tension pneumothorax is an important reversible cause of cardiac arrest.

Answer 8:

4) Pulseless electrical activity: shocking the patient stops all cardiac activity. This is useful in fast, disorganized rhythms, which can be stopped in the hope that a slower rhythm will emerge afterwards. Pulseless electrical activity is therefore not amenable to shocking.

Answer 9:

5) Pulseless ventricular tachycardia: the ventricles are contracting in fast, uncoordinated fashion, allowing no cardiac output. Shocking can stop this cycle, slowing down contractions and allowing cardiac output to increase.

Answer 10:

4) Pulseless electrical activity: this is the definition of pulseless electrical activity.

ADVANCED LIFE SUPPORT: SBAs

Answer 11:

2) Adrenaline 1 mg intravenously: adrenaline is given intravenously and not intramuscularly (IM) in cardiac arrest as IM would not reach the circulation because of the lack of perfusion. Asystole is a non-shockable rhythm.

Index

Note: Page numbers with brackets e.g. 211–14(220–3), are to questions with the answer indicated in brackets.

Anaesthesia

Anaesthesia

Anaesthesia

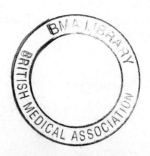